Palgrave Texts in Counselling and Psychotherapy

Series Editors
Arlene Vetere
Family Therapy and Systemic Practice
VID Specialized University
Oslo, Norway

Rudi Dallos
Clinical Psychology
Plymouth University
Plymouth, UK

This series introduces readers to the theory and practice of counselling and psychotherapy across a wide range of topical issues. Ideal for both trainees and practitioners, the books will appeal to anyone wishing to use counselling and psychotherapeutic skills and will be particularly relevant to workers in health, education, social work and related settings. The books in this series emphasise an integrative orientation weaving together a variety of models including, psychodynamic, attachment, trauma, narrative and systemic ideas. The books are written in an accessible and readable style with a focus on practice. Each text offers theoretical background and guidance for practice, with creative use of clinical examples.

Arlene Vetere, Professor of Family Therapy and Systemic Practice at VID Specialized University, Oslo, Norway.

Rudi Dallos, Emeritus Professor, Dept. of Clinical Psychology, University of Plymouth, UK.

More information about this series at
http://www.palgrave.com/gp/series/16540

Vivienne Purcell

Understanding Visible Differences

Working Therapeutically With Individuals Who Look Different

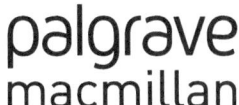

Vivienne Purcell
Lyndhurst, Hampshire, UK

ISSN 2662-9127 ISSN 2662-9135 (electronic)
Palgrave Texts in Counselling and Psychotherapy
ISBN 978-3-030-51654-3 ISBN 978-3-030-51655-0 (eBook)
https://doi.org/10.1007/978-3-030-51655-0

Cover illustration: Flavio Coelho/gettyimages

This Palgrave Macmillan imprint is published by the registered company Springer Nature Switzerland AG.
The registered company address is: Gewerbestrasse 11, 6330 Cham, Switzerland

Author's note—all comments attributed to interviewees have been viewed and approved by them prior to publication. All case examples and material used to facilitate understanding of issues have been anonymised and do not refer to identifiable clinical cases.

Acknowledgements

I have written this book as a resource for supervisors, therapists, their clients and those caring others who wish to understand more. It is intended to be a brief and wide-ranging work to complement those specialist reference books which are excellent clinical resources. It is the one I often wished for in busy supervision sessions.

The generous contributions of interviewees who were willing to share their own experiences of caring for, adjusting to and living with difference have been invaluable. I'd like to thank Jo Williams, Kenny Ardouin, Beth Angella, Sasha Lynne, Kay Kay, Paul McSharry and Beth Shaw in particular, for their time and openness. Their approval was sought for all interview comments used prior to publication.

Finally, huge thanks to Arlene Vetere, Rudi Dallos, Mike and Kit Neill whose help, belief and encouragement I have been able to rely on.

An Overview: 'Naming and Fear'

Even in a multicultural society most people have little difficulty in recognising others whose physical appearance is outside the norm. Historically human social groups are formed by blood ties which amplify and assign value to recognised similarities and geographic interests, and appearance is an important signifier of 'people like us', often reinforced by marriage/partnership patterns (Berry 2000). Favoured and disfavoured characteristics within social groups are to some extent historically/socially formed, and as such are mediated by status and variable over time, but also impacted by the resources and survival needs of the group. Tradition matters, and normalises beliefs and behaviours. Mary Douglas, in her early anthropological work *Purity and Danger* (1966), studied how these patterned beliefs maintain symbolic boundaries in ritual, religion and lifestyle.

It does not take much imagination to realise that a person with physical differences outside the normal range and/or limitations may frequently confer fewer advantages on a small isolated human group. Such differences may be tolerated more easily in an adult (say) who is injured in battle but has knowledge and/or wisdom to share, than a dependent child. Female, and to a lesser extent male, children whose marriageability is affected by physical defects are also more likely to be regarded as liabilities or sources of shame in honour-based cultures.

Historically in many traditional societies infants or adults that looked different at birth would be ostracised or killed, with superstitious beliefs associated to them, such as fearing they would bring bad luck, and there are examples today of communities which regard having a different or disabled child as shaming. The African Child Policy Forum (ACPF) (2011) based on field studies in Cameroon, Ethiopia, Senegal, Uganda and Zambia concluded that 'common beliefs about the causes of child-hood disability include: sin or promiscuity of the mother, an ancestral curse; or demonic possession' (Eskay et al. 2012). The prospects for such children and their mothers can be very bleak, particularly in groups with limited resources. More hopefully in Nigeria there has been a public edu-cation campaign and dissemination of disability-related information with the intention of overcoming persistent false beliefs about disability. These previously included a curse from God, ancestral violations of social norms, offences against the local Gods, witches and wizard actions, adul-tery and more.

These beliefs may at first seem outlandish, but in the UK the discovery of disability during pregnancy frequently results in a termination where there are no strong counter beliefs. For example, 63% of foetuses identi-fied with spina bifida and 83% of those with anencephaly were aborted (Johnson et al. 2012). Few loving parents would choose a disability for their child, and they are encouraged to 'try again' by doctors, hoping for one that is able-bodied, clever and beautiful, or at least average.

In all cases stigmatising messages and behaviours aimed at individuals or minorities create anxiety and avoidance which may be experienced at a group, family and individual level. Those who look different report a routine loss of privacy caused by staring and personal comments, which can be very aversive. Exposure to aversive experiences without under-standing, support and help to manage these interactions creates psycho-logical distress. Without this, fearful predictions of similar upsetting experiences in future social interactions can result in a pattern of low self-esteem, shame and associated negative feelings and behaviours, limit-ing the interactions and opportunities of those who have been stigmatised.

For clinical work to succeed there must be sufficient therapeutic alli-ance to permit focus on these internalised thoughts and feelings, without reactivating shame, so that over time the individual expands their social network and comes to believe that any ignorance and prejudice they encounter are the problem of the other, rather than internalising it. They also need to acquire skill and understanding in social interactions to manage the natural curiosity of others when they encounter difference.

References

African Child Policy Forum (2011) Violence against children with disabilities in Africa: field studies. Cameroon, Ethiopia, Senegal, Uganda and Zambia

Berry DS (2000) Attractiveness, attraction, and sexual selection: Evolutionary perspectives on the form and function of physical attractiveness. Advances in Experimental Social Psychology 32:273–342. Elsevier

Douglas M (1966) Purity and dange*r: an analysis of concepts of pollution and taboo*. Routledge and Keegan Paul

Eskay M, Onu VC, Igbo JN, Obiyo N, Ugwuanyi L (2012) Disability within the African Culture 478, University of Nigeria, Nsukka, US-China Education Review B2. Source: www.un.org-socdev-disability. Toolkit on Disability for Africa

Johnson C et al (2012) Pregnancy termination following prenatal diagnosis of anencephaly or spina bifidia: a systematic review of clinical literature. Birth Defects Research Part A Clinical Molecular Teratology 94(11):857–863

Contents

1   What Do We Mean by 'Visible Difference'?   1

2   The Social Construction of Difference and Disability   11

3   The Developing Self: The Differences of Difference   33

4   The Family Context   59

5   Relationships: Outside of the Family Group   77

6   Assessment and Treatment Planning   95

7   Healing Conversations   115

8   Thinking About Treatment Plans and Models: A Formulation-Based Approach   131

Some Final Thoughts   155

Appendix: Brief Summary of Types of Visible Difference   159

Resources Support and Information   169

Index   175

List of Figures

Fig. 8.1   Factors for treatment plans   132

Fig. 8.2   CBT basic formulation example   135

Fig. 8.3   Three areas formulation diagram   137

Fig. 8.4   Diagram adapted from Lee (2009)   142

Fig. 8.5   Anita's 'Bottom Line' (schema, core belief) global negative self-judgement (or feared truth). Adapted from Lee (2009)   152

List of Tables

Table 8.1   Her treatment diagram looked something like this   143
Table 8.2   His treatment diagram looked like this—(20+ sessions) TBA   147

1

What Do We Mean by 'Visible Difference'?

A Story

Grownups often said what a lovely brave boy Jack was. He didn't really know why. The children at school said different things—'what's wrong with your face?' or 'weirdo', or some other stupid thing. Sometimes a few of them called names, pretended 'it' was catching, screamed and ran away, then said it was just a game. Especially if he had been in hospital for some surgery on his face and the swelling hadn't completely gone. Though Jack was used to how he looked even he thought he was a bit scary weird then. Teachers usually stopped the game when they found out, eventually. Once, during circle time at Whitegates Primary, Mr. Davies talked about the ways that people could be different and what it meant, and Jack had a chance to explain his difference and how he was born that way which helped. Luckily, another girl in the class talked about her difference too, which was a relief. Then she wanted to hang out with Jack all the time, but she was a bit annoying so he tried to avoid her. He felt sorry when she cried, but also fed up that everyone thought they should play together because they were both different. There was more to friendship than that he thought! Usually he made one or two friends, never any of

© The Author(s) 2020
V. Purcell, *Understanding Visible Differences*, Palgrave Texts in Counselling and
Psychotherapy, https://doi.org/10.1007/978-3-030-51655-0_1

the really popular people, but there were always a few odd ones in every class, quiet or sad or awkward. Or just smarter than everyone else. They were more interesting and they got used to him. His dad was in the army, so he had been to a few schools and knew how to get by, act tough when he needed to. When things were really bad, he found ways to be on his own, reading, playing games, making things, or out in the wilds if he could find any.

He was in the last year of primary now, and due to go to secondary school in the autumn. Things had got better here over time, and everyone in the class seemed OK with him mostly. Jack and his friend Nick liked to play in the fields behind the houses, which led all the way up to the woods at the top. From there they could see far away to Oxford sometimes, and watch the kites circling in the thermals. Both of them loved birds, and Nick's dad worked at the bird sanctuary. It was here he learned how to hold them on his arm in the field, release their hoods and let them fly. It was the most fantastic feeling he knew, even better than running and shouting in the dark on the way home. He felt his heart lift with them and imagined what it was like to soar free above everything. Getting them to return to the lure was a bond, a connection to something wild. It was a safe place.

Like his dog Jessie, the birds didn't care what Jack looked like, it was just about trust and heart and fun. He thought that was probably a kind of true love because his mum and dad often said the way he looked didn't matter, and not to mind when people said silly things. Mum said that when people get to know you they see who you really are. That made sense to Jack, because with every operation he looked a bit different. He thought one day the surgeons might make him look normal, which would be a relief though it shouldn't matter.

Generally, Jack was fine. There were just a few things that really bothered him. Like never being picked for the football team, when he thought some of the others who got picked regularly weren't as good. Nick was often picked, but he deserved it and Jack went to games to cheer him on. Sam, who was always in the team liked the glory, but Nick worked incessantly to set up the shots and made him look good. That was the way things seemed to work, Jack thought, some people had it easy.

It was Saturday evening, Jack was propped up on his bed, the room was quiet, but he was in turmoil, thinking back over the events of the last couple of days, trying to work out exactly how things had changed. Also playing Morrowind in a slightly distracted way, his eyes misting over when he thought about certain things, making it hard to see the screen. He always played this game when he wanted to be somewhere else in his head. He was a prince now with territories to defend.

This Friday at football practice was pretty much like all the others. Jack had enjoyed the game, scored a couple, wasn't picked. But on Saturday morning the phone rang. Dad answered, and Jack heard him say, 'I'm sure it will be fine. He can look after himself.' He put the phone down, came into the kitchen where Jack was still eating the pancakes Mum liked to cook on Saturdays and said 'Sam has twisted his knee, so you're on the team for this afternoon's friendly match at Marlow. If you like.' Mum made a face at Dad and said 'you know how rough those games can be' trailing off. Dad looked at her, then Jack, and said 'do you want to?' 'Yes!' he shouted, running up the stairs to get his kit. Dad followed and said more quietly 'Don't do anything that would worry your mum'. Jack knew what he was talking about, and just shrugged. 'I'm always careful'. Mum worried about him falling, or being in a rumble, getting hit or something that would mean more surgery.

They arrived at the club with just enough time to get ready. Running out, Jack felt a bit weird to be actually on the pitch, instead of watching with the others. Mostly family of people playing. Nick's sister Kate was there, chatting to Chloe, Ted, Josh and a few others. Dad of course. Mr. Gates the team coach finished his talk with 'Just do your best boys' and everyone ran out. The whistle went, and once they started running and passing it felt like being back on the pitch at school, only more intense, more surprising. The other team were pushing hard, but Jack felt confident they had them. Nick and he fell into a rhythm, passing between them up the pitch, the goal was open, and Jack scored. Yay!!! Huge cheers, and in the corner of his eye saw Dad going mad on the side, taking photos. The others clapped Jack on the back, hugged, and he considered trying a triumphal knee skid, but decided not. The game was on again, and the others were trying even harder to get a goal back now. Jack's team were doing well, lining another one up, but Ted slipped on the mud and it bounced off the bar. On and on, as each team struggled to keep the ball out of their end and attack the goal.

At half time they were 1–0, feeling tired, but still determined to win. Running out again for the second half they were all convinced they could do it. Jack didn't know quite how it happened, but the other side seemed to find a gap really quickly and suddenly it was 1–1. They were triumphant, and now Jack's team could see them pushing harder. They had to do something! Nick and Ted set off towards their goal, passing tightly between them, the Ted to Jack, Jack to Nick, now in a sweet spot, and he put it in like a professional. A goal worthy of a knee skid, they had pulled it back. They needed another one to be safe though, and they struggled on through a second half which seemed much longer than the first, never quite getting the ball in, but neither did the other side. Just before the whistle Nick passed Jack a sweet cross, a space opened, and the ball was in. Everyone on their side erupted in hysterical cheers, they heard the final high-pitched screech, and it was all over. The other team trudged despondently off the pitch, but they were surrounded by their cheering friends and family, with the Dads looking as if they had scored the goals themselves. Jack was not used to this, not quite sure how to handle it, but felt fantastic at the same time. Even the girls looked at him differently he thought, and Kate said 'you were really great, I didn't know you could play like that'. 'Neither did I' said Jack, blushing slightly, and the girls laughed as they turned away. As they walked off he heard Chloe say 'He fancies you! I bet he would ask you out if he could. Poor you, what would you say?' And laughed teasingly. Kate said 'Don't be like that' and then Chloe ran off shouting 'You do too, you do', with Kate following 'not him!'

Jack watched them, suddenly feeling as if someone had slipped a small blade between his ribs, a stabbing, shaming pain.

Back in his room, turning it over again in his mind while battering a few monsters in Morrowind, he decided he wouldn't go to the leaving disco after all. The only problem was how to explain it to Mum and Dad.

How We Define Differences Makes a Difference

Jack is a regular young boy, with some unusual experiences. He isn't average in appearance and probably will never be, though at this age he may well think that one day the surgeons will pull off the final miracle. He's not hoping for good looks, just normal. Of course, like the rest of us, he might not be satisfied with that!

It will not be until he becomes a young adult he will really 'get' that it probably won't happen and he will have to live his whole life being different. Generally, this is the toughest time.

From this brief story the reader will note that Jack has already had a lot of experience of being different and come to some conclusions about what it means for him. These have come naturally, and like all our heuristics and biases have developed as a result of experiences. Some people have it easy. He is less likely to be picked. Being too different is risky. People can be thoughtless and cruel. He is resilient, and has learned how to find ways to soothe himself when things go wrong. He doesn't always share his hurt and disappointment, working out what he wants to do on his own.

> Jack is about to make a choice to withdraw from an important event for fear of being hurt and shamed, and this could become a pattern. Imagine meeting Jack as a client in 10 years time. How easy do you think it will be to access these complex chains of experiences and decisions? How likely is it that he will remember?

Jack is visibly different and able bodied. 'Visibly Different' is a relatively new descriptor for people that in earlier times might have been described as 'deformed' or 'disfigured' in face and/or body and one intended to be value-neutral. This quite recent change shows an increased awareness, sensitivity and concern about the impact of naming. Not all activists agree with it, believing that previous crueller, excluding terms are a more accurate reflection of the judgements of 'normal' society which needs to be confronted, not finessed away. Within the category of 'visible difference' there is huge diversity. Someone could be registered blind but otherwise able bodied, or a wheelchair user with a beautiful face, or the opposite. Each person's experience and medical journey will be unlike most other people's. Being born different is a world away from becoming different, having been 'normal', and this must be considered as part of any attempt to understand lived experiences.

From a medical/professional point of view I have listed in the Appendix the main forms of visible difference the reader is likely to encounter. Please remember that these are categories of professional convenience to some extent. Each 'category' contains a diversity of presentation and severity. Many now have charities associated with them and I have gathered the main ones in the 'Resources, Support and Information' section at the end of the book.

About This Book

The material offered here covers a lot of ground, some of which may be less relevant to your current interest. Feel free to 'skip' to the chapters which attract you first. This may initially be the Chap. 8 case studies if you have a current client in your clinic that you want to do better with. Or possibly Chaps. 6 and 7 if you recognise a need to improve the therapeutic relationship and communication. As an experienced practitioner you may find the discussion of different therapeutic stances and models very brief, particularly in relation to your preferred approach. References are offered for those less familiar with some approaches who want to delve deeper. I hope it will be useful to the integrative practitioner, as well as those required to work mainly in one model, inviting consideration of a flexible method (within competence). This material has also been included to assist the curious reader less familiar with the technology of therapy. It is hoped that more experienced readers will also find something to stimulate a new approach.

Chapters 2, 3, 4, and 5 will be useful when you want to understand more about the context of your client's development. They are important because they will assist your reflections on the lived experience of someone who is born with or acquires visible differences.

The impact of our pervasive sociocultural context is considered in Chap. 2. It begins with a brief overview of how longstanding attitudes are both established and mitigated through accepted norms and cultural production. It then invites you to consider the way that younger generations are using social media platforms to challenge narrative biases which were all-pervasive in earlier decades. The chapter is structured to include 'think boxes' with questions or suggested resources to stimulate your understanding and clinical work. Chapters 3, 4, and 5 explore some of the research relating to development and visible difference, the family context, and developing and managing relationships outside of the (hopefully supportive) family group. These are offered to deepen your understanding of potential difficulties at different stages, which your client may not associate with current presenting issues.

Where Does Psychological Therapy Fit In?

It is important for the therapist to have sufficient understanding of their client's condition, and some awareness of the range of possible impact. But one of the potential weaknesses of the 'typological' approach when planning psychological therapy is that it can create unhelpful assumptions and expectations in the therapist about their client's concerns and distress. At the point of assessment their presenting problem may be unrelated or have a tangential relationship to their visible difference. If there are useful connections to be made, this needs to happen at the most helpful and acceptable moment for the client. A blunt and clumsy attempt to make a connection may feel stigmatising and cause your client to feel that the therapy agenda is not shared. However, the association may be there, as part of the individual's whole orientation to the world, or self-concept, and it is helpful to have this in mind as a possibility for future reflection.

This underlines the importance of history taking as part of the assessment process, and the creation of materials, for instance a genogram and timeline, which can be revisited later if needed.

One useful question is whether the client has been offered or had therapy as part of their hospital or outpatient experience. The answer may depend on their age at the time of treatment—if it was a congenital condition counselling or therapy may have been offered to the parents not the child in the first instance. Their current age is also a factor, as the understanding that psychological support is necessary for good adjustment has not reliably been supported with funding in the UK. In 2020 the offer of therapy services differs between presentations and is very restricted. Specialist therapy services, where they exist, are most usually found in a hospital outpatient setting and are not evenly spread throughout the country.

The real process of ongoing adjustment and understanding will be very different for someone with a congenital defect, compared with the person who suffers a traumatic shock and leaves hospital visibly different. In both cases though, the ongoing psychological work to achieve an accepting and self-actualising identity will occur post discharge. Most likely it will be a process of change through many discharges and life stages.

Erving Goffman in his very early work on stigma (1963) suggests that visible markings define a person as 'spoiled' and therefore less attractive and valued by others. He describes shame as central to the experience of stigma. This cruel truth is played out most clearly in the person who was relatively happy with their appearance prior to a traumatic event, and leaves hospital after treatment at odds with an unacceptable new image in the mirror. The frequent response is 'I just can't be this person', an indicator of possible psychological risk. Moving away from their own internalised fear of difference, which they may not have been aware of, and rebuilding their identity is the challenge of a lifetime.

Kent and Thompson (2002) suggest that shame is likely to pay a crucial role in adjustment to disfigurement drawing on Fredrickson and Robert's 'Objectification theory' (1997) which will be considered further in the chapter on Assessment and Treatment planning. David Veale describes a similar model which he uses to explain the maintaining patterns of body dysmorphic disorder, selective attention and rumination. This processing of self as a spoiled aesthetic object maintains distress.

While this process is as relevant to those working with enduring visible difference, there is an obvious difference between this group and those with dysmorphia. People suffering the very real psychological distress of body dysmorphia have the potential to recover and recognise themselves as within the normal range, acceptable to themselves and others. Those with enduring visible differences need to construct their identity and self-worth around different criteria, developing new life skills to manage prejudice when they encounter it. This is the rationale for focusing this work on visible differences, while recognising the impact of social and media pressures on those with appearance anxiety who may be regarded by others as being within the 'norms'.

The clinician needs to remain mindful that prejudice can be real and not minimise, and the person affected needs to acquire skills in how to manage this and connect with support of others in a way they find helpful. The increasing number of online resources and groups available makes this a potential source of immediate support. Older people who may never have met others like themselves growing up are less likely to have had access to these. This once again highlights the importance of working over time to change the social discourse, and decrease the isolating effects of shame.

References

Fredrickson BL, Roberts TA (1997) Toward understanding women's lived experiences and mental health risks. Psychology of Women Quarterly Wiley Online Library

Goffman E (1963) Stigma: notes on the management of spoiled identity. Penguin Books

Kent G, Thompson AR (2002) Models of disfigurement: implications for treatment. In: Gilbert P, Miles J (eds) Understanding body shame. Brunner-Routledge, Hove, pp 106–116

2

The Social Construction of Difference and Disability

Throughout the history of human communities there have always been people whose appearance and capacities deviated from the socially accepted 'normal', due to genetic variation, disease and accident. Though many of those unable to function independently would have been killed, we know from the fossil history that some (with both congenital and acquired difference) survived into adulthood. We also know that some were protected by high status and their disabilities erased from public images, as the pharaohs Tutankhamun who had a club foot, and the Mummy 61074 which has an elongated skull, cleft palate and prominent cheekbones show. There is vigorous speculation that these are the remains of Akhenaten.

In contrast, in the same region Seneb c252, whose dwarfism is depicted, was able to be an architect with status, as dwarfism was not regarded as a defect. The dwarf god Bes, protector of childbirth, humour, music and dancing, was very popular. However, in Seneb's tomb his family statue was made with the couple sitting, emphasising their similarities. In other societies, for instance Medieval France, the high-status person's acquired disability might be accepted because of their position. Charles VI of France inherited his throne aged 11 in the middle of the Hundred Years War. He was given the epithet of 'the Beloved' when he came to maturity

© The Author(s) 2020
V. Purcell, *Understanding Visible Differences*, Palgrave Texts in Counselling and
Psychotherapy, https://doi.org/10.1007/978-3-030-51655-0_2

and gained power. It later changed in popular use to 'the Mad' when his psychotic episodes became more visible, florid and frequent.[1]

In more recent times the perception of fitness to govern has become sensitive to physical appearances. Franklin D. Roosevelt successfully cultivated the image of a healthy man who had recovered from polio with no significant disability, though this was not the case (Brune and Wilson 2013). This mattered to his political ambitions. The act of 'passing' was achieved with the complicity of press and advisers over many years. In fact, he could only walk with difficulty and spent most of his time in a wheelchair or sitting. In the Democratic conventions of 1924 and 1928 he was determined not to be wheeled in. He achieved this after much practice with the help of his son James, who supported him to his seat before the delegates arrived. No press photos of him in a wheelchair were permitted. His apparent achievements were presented to other polio survivors as a role model by doctors, therapists, family and friends, though they were not realistic. Roosevelt had a team of people managing his image and ensuring that he was able to access buildings and rooms. The important message conveyed to other sufferers was that by minimising the extent of disability it was possible to 'pass' in normal society and avoid stigma (Brune and Wilson 2013).

What do you think the psychological cost of 'passing' is? Most of the writing on this lived experience is about race—see 'Passing for White' by James M. O'Toole (2003) University of Massachusetts Press. But 'Passing for Normal' by Amy S. Wilensky (2000 Broadway Books) explores the author's experience of growing up with Tourette's and OCD, feeling like a 'freak'.

How Do We Construct Meaning Around Difference?

Falvey (2012) states 'culture can be described … as referring to the system of shared beliefs, meanings, values, patterns of behaviour, customs and artefacts with which members of a society identify and use in coping with one another and the world'.

---

[1] This example of an emerging mental health disorder falls outside the main definition of visible differences. Unusually, Charles VI's disorder was highly visible, unlike many who were mentally ill at this time, and is included for this reason.

As previously noted, evolutionary psychologists argue that where appearance is concerned social variation is constrained by deep and intrinsic associations between physical appearance and biological correlates. In more recent times these continue to be understood as important for mate selection and healthy reproduction. Converging standards of beauty may be in the ascendant across societies, despite concerns about discrimination towards ethnic differences. While status is still a mediator, some argue that this is increasingly true in the current period of globalised communication. Researchers continue to find corresponding assessments of attractiveness and valued physical traits across cultures, fanned by social media (Shaffer et al. 2000, Orbach 2009 and Widdows 2018).

The social constructionist perspective sees ideas about the social world as something created through interchange with others, rather than existing as a 'given' external reality (Gergen 1985). To illustrate this Gergen cites the concept of childhood, which was not always considered a special phase of development, the idea of romantic love, and the individualistic concept of the self as examples of this process of production and change. Recently ubiquitous in Western societies, some of these ideas are being contrasted by the traditions of migrant communities with different histories. The outcome of this co-existence remains to be seen, but we can easily find examples of parallel value systems and different human outcomes in contemporary UK society. Possibly efforts to become a more integrated community are encouraging an interrogation of social assumptions. We can hope that any discriminatory practices are being challenged across all communities, and this will include definitions and valuing of difference. But it can be slow going. The current shift in the social perception of disabled athletes marks a change in the 'map of the territory' (Bateson 2002) in some ways. But so far, they are 'exceptions'. Many who are visibly different will still recount stories of bullying, abuse or unthinking discrimination. So there are good reasons for wishing to 'pass' if you can.

Learning to Live with and Challenge the Meaning of Difference

Included in the idea of social construction is the understanding that these complex constructed meanings require multiple actors, individuals or groups. These may have preconceptions, anxieties and/or negative assumptions about the other, and differences in power. Analysis of these competing forces helps us to understand how meaning and value are produced. It hardly needs to be said that those who have more power, particularly the cultural power to define, have usually controlled the production and meaning of information through words and images. It is still true that these complex networks of meaning are often experienced as 'given' by vulnerable individuals, especially as they move through the education system.

It is not easy for someone born into any system of meaning to perceive it as other than the 'natural order' without help, and then understand how to challenge it, especially if it disadvantages while defining them. The history of women's suffrage in the UK shows that if not completely necessary then it is very helpful for the individual defined as having an inferior status to join with similar others. Through exchange the opportunity arises to create new perspectives, finding ways to articulate those thoughts and feelings left out of current definitions. Then it may be a long struggle (depending on your aims!). For someone wishing to redefine their understanding of themselves the process of therapy might be a beginning, or some stage in this journey. Alongside this, although social media has increased the victimisation of some people, it has also created the opportunity for groups of similar people to connect with each other, share experiences and realise they are not alone. The stereotypes of 'difference' can be challenged for the first time, without permission from a powerful social actor, and the voices of individuals can gain a media following. From this platform changed attitudes and beliefs can become the 'new normal'.

> But not everyone wants to be a social warrior, nor should they be obliged to explain their difference if they are not in the mood. Though the loss of privacy which comes with difference can make it difficult to politely decline intrusive questioning.

Therapy as a Safe Space to Consider Change

Social change still takes time, even if the timescale has been reduced, and protective patterns of thought and behaviour may be well established through long experience.

In new social contexts clients anticipating they may be discriminated against may habitually be very cautious, withdraw or avoid. The other parties who fear making a mistake and causing offence may do the same, perpetuating the experience of isolation and accompanying belief systems. This can happen in a therapeutic context like any other, and can feel frustrating if the therapist is working to create a therapeutic alliance. But each situation also offers the opportunity to challenge and alter the pattern in a safe environment, and caution can be noted and wondered about in a way that will later be helpful. Think about how you would try to approach this dilemma.

This is a topic I will return to, with a consideration of the mentalisation-based approach when working with young people in particular.

Reflection could lead later to an exploration of the usefulness and constraints of the person's habitual approach, opening an interest in experimentation. As part of the therapist's toolkit this is one purpose of social skills training which might give the affected person the opportunity to feel more in control of new social encounters through active explanation. This may be the first time that they are able to successfully manage their own and to some extent other people's interpretation of a situation. A recent (2020) report on Sky news features Tulsi Vagjani, who was 10 when a family holiday to India led to tragedy. Her parents and younger brother were killed in a plane crash and she was left with severe facial burns. Now aged 30 she details her experience of bullying at school once she left hospital, and later on discrimination in finding a job, saying '*I don't get to take off my scars*'. She describes '*One of the worst experiences was when I was waiting at a bus stop. This car came along with 4 guys in, they opened the window and shouted "you deserve to die because you're so +++ing ugly".*' This devastated her social confidence as a young woman, understandably. Having received support, she now speaks as part of a campaign to raise awareness, as well as being a Pilates instructor. Now aged 30 she says '*it's not normal and not acceptable, and people should know that these types of things can be reported as a hate crime.'* This recognition of prejudice and discrimination as a social problem, not a personal failing, can be liberating.

The Social Experience of Self

Commentators point out that in well-functioning able-bodied experience the body is largely un-noticed, whereas someone with a functional impairment experiences the world through their disability, especially in an environment mainly designed for the able bodied. Marginalisation is built-in.

> To test out this assertion just imagine the not un-stressful experience of getting to the airport and catching your flight, then re-imagine it in a wheelchair. How would it alter your attitudes to travel, and levels of anxiety? How might you begin a conversation about this if you thought it was relevant to your client?

This is a crucial difference, and very important to hold in mind during clinical assessment as it may impact how the individual experiences themselves in relation to others in important ways. The wheelchair-bound person has a marginalised but stable social experience on the underground. Someone who has difficulties in movement, speech, sight or an equivalent will experience the world through their disability. It is not something that can easily be forgotten as there are constant reminders in an ableist society. In a new encounter they are more likely to be aware that the other person has noticed they are different.

In contrast, someone who looks different but functions as 'able bodied' may experience themselves as 'normal' unless they are disabled socially by others' attitudes. It can be forgotten (by them) when moving through the world, while being obvious to others. Meeting them for the first time requires a performance from the unacquainted other, which the person with a visible difference may be unaware of. Or it may be badly done, creating self-conscious awkwardness on both sides. While the challenges for the functionally normal person may appear (and are) far fewer, there is the possibility of misunderstanding and concealed prejudice. There is also a (largely unrecognised) issue for those who have a concealed or invisible difference. While this is not the focus of this book, it is something for the therapist to bear in mind, especially during assessment.

Once again, if this is potentially relevant to your client, mentally role-play how you might open up this issue in a helpful way

Exploring the Construction of Difference and Stigma in Media in a Therapy Context

Social construction and comparison theories allow the opportunity to explore the influences on current thinking about appearance and identity, making links with production of identities in film and media, which are a helpful guide to current mainstream values of a given culture. This is a complex and densely theorised field, but nevertheless once the basic mechanisms are understood the lay person can more easily perceive distortions in representations, as current social media discussions on the representations of ethnicity, sexuality and gender testify.

These are all groups which have at one time suffered in accordance with Goffman's (1963) definition of stigma in which he identifies three types 'First there are the abominations of the body—the various physical deformities. Next there are the blemishes of character perceived as weak will, domineering or unnatural passions, treacherous and rigid beliefs, and dishonesty, these being inferred from a known record of, for example, mental disorder, imprisonment, addiction, alcoholism, homosexuality, unemployment, suicidal attempts, and radical political behaviour. Finally, there are the tribal stigma of race, nation, and religion, these being stigma that transmit through lineages and equally contaminate all members of a family ... he (sic) possesses a stigma, an undesired differentness from what we had anticipated. We and those who do not depart negatively from the particular expectations at issue I shall call the "normals".'

Such use of language today would probably get Goffman both fired and stigmatised, and it comes as a shock to realise that his cold-eyed social analysis is not entirely irrelevant now, even if the wording is. Both you and your client inhabit a world saturated with implicit values and exploring these through the common ground of favourite soap operas, films or music can facilitate reflection on feelings and fears otherwise hard to access. It may require a bit of homework from you, but can move the therapy work on and facilitate a better therapeutic relationship.

The media representations of difference and 'normalness' that accompanied Goffman's analysis have been more thoroughly explored by academics since his time, creating a space to work for change. The under-representation of all women (Tuchman 1979) was understood to reflect their lack of power and status in society. This is still a focus of women's activism. Other sub-groups, like older people, minorities, the disabled and visibly different, were and are under-represented. This can be cumulative. So, an older, low income, disabled woman from a minority group might suffer from multiple disadvantages. Commentators also highlighted the way that stereotypical portrayals of men in popular films like the 'Die Hard' series, Lethal Weapon, Robocop and so on typically show men as aggressive, dominant, unafraid, violent, lacking emotions and emphatically not feminine (Wood 1994). A tricky performance to pull off if you happen to be in a wheelchair, though the television series 'Ironside' starring Raymond Burr (previously Perry Mason) depicts him in a wheelchair after being shot. Aired between 1967 and 1975 it began during the period of the Vietnam War for the USA, when many soldiers returned with serious injuries. This arguably fits with the hypermasculine narrative, now beginning to be challenged by gender-neutral identities.

If you have a client who has clearly been the victim of several forms of discrimination in the past (or currently), how would you engage them in thinking about how social representation impacts on their daily life? How would you avoid a further negative impact, or unhelpful emphasis of difference between you and your client? What do you think about sharing your own experiences in this context (if relevant)?

'Toby's Room' a book by Pat Barker (2012) uses the First World War to consider the transformations and disruptions of relationships in wartime. She describes vividly the horrific facial injuries suffered by soldiers, their psychological distress, social rejection and the pioneering work done by surgeons at Queens Hospital, near London. Henry Tonks' drawings of this work are available to view online at http://www.gilliesarchives.org.uk together with photographs and case histories of some patients. This is still a very useful archive for therapists attempting to understand aspects of their client's medical journey.

Sometimes film and television media dramatise and normalise social attitudes. Fear of different others was dramatised in 'The Invasion of the Body Snatchers' (1956) in which a homespun Californian town is invaded by seed pod aliens who can replicate every aspect of a human being except their emotions (they don't feel like us). They can also be subtle agents of change—after being used as a textbook example for cultural studies students, it was later satirised in 'District 9' (2009) which explores themes of xenophobia and social segregation.

The original Hunchback of Notre Dame film (1932) is based on Victor Hugo's 1831 novel in which the deformed hunchback Quasimodo is instructed to capture the gypsy Esmerelda. Paul Longmore (2003) argues that this original characterisation of the sex starved and criminal disabled 'monster', depicts disabled people not as a social minority with civil rights but as victims of a tragic fate, '*The depiction of the disabled person as a monster and the criminal characterization both express to varying degrees the notion that disability involves the loss of an essential part of one's humanity. Depending on the extent of the disability, the individual is perceived as more or less subhuman.*'

Disney's cartoon retelling of the same story (1996) is more subtle and complex, mapping and to a certain extent leading the way in a shift in social attitudes by encouraging empathy in young viewers. It shows Quasimodo as the epitome of disability, playing with dolls, hidden away by the cruel Minister of Justice Judge Claude Frollo, who is charged with his care, but instead isolates him in the bell-tower with only gargoyles as friends. He is taken out at the 'Festival of Fools' and labelled the 'King of Fools' for having the ugliest face in Paris. But in this telling the 'baddie' is the 'normal looking' villain Frollo who behaves as the monster. In the end Quasimodo is the hero who saves Esmerelda and receives her acceptance and kindness in return. The children viewing the story are invited to identify with Esmerelda (or Quasimodo). This seems a good thing, but Nelson (1994) notes how this struggle transforms him into someone amazing rather than just ordinary, and how this process often belittles 'ordinary' people with disabilities. He doesn't get the girl either, and even in the Disney retelling of the fable 'Beauty and the Beast', the beast must transform into a handsome prince for a truly happy ending.

These examples from popular culture are very useful to therapists, showing examples of moments when a culture can be observed 'correcting' earlier prejudices. For someone who is different though, the opposite experience can happen, when prejudices assumed to be part of the past suddenly present themselves as very much alive and kicking.

This happened to me a few years ago when I went to see a film called 'Men and Chicken (2015 Danish comedy)'. The review sounded promising, and we hoped for an evening of offbeat humour. It definitely provided that! The hero of the tale was a university lecturer who had returned to visit his three brothers, because there were some problems in the local village. The brothers all lived in a rambling property inherited from the father, who was a scientist. While he was alive, he worked on a mysterious 'project'. None of the brothers remembered a mother, but had grown up together, with little outside contact. The central 'joke' was that they all had cleft repairs alongside other deformities, as an indicator of their 'difference' and were getting into trouble locally with clumsy Frankenstein-type attempts to relate to local women. The more 'normal' lecturer-brother (who had social skills) had to attempt to resolve the ensuing problems as chaos and violence escalated. None of them knew much about their father's work, but they kept chickens which they had a special bond with. It later transpired as the situation unspooled that their deformities were caused by the father's genetic 'experiments' in which he had created human-animal hybrids. Hence the title. This description sounds so awful I must say again that it was quite funny in parts. But so, so, unacceptably wrong in so many ways that I was completely gob-smacked. I really couldn't believe that such a script had been approved in twenty-first-century Europe. At the end I walked out of the cinema in a state of shock and said to my companion 'what just happened?' He (with no visible difference) had the same reaction.

Your client may have similar experiences to share.

From 'Difference' to Discrimination: A Very Short History and Journey

This social construction of meaning around appearance includes aspects of ethnicity which can trigger vulnerability to 'appearance related distress' in a minority through migration to an area where they are visibly different to the dominant group and encounter prejudice. The accounts of early migrants to the UK in the 1960s (Goffman's era), where they encountered signs like 'no blacks, no Irish, no dogs', bear this out, and the painful difficulties for their children in mainly white schools. The early struggle for civil rights was a defining part of the shift in social attitudes in the 1960s and encouraged disability rights campaigns at the same time.

Both continue, and even in twenty-first century parents on social media and news sites discuss how to cope with their children starting school and wishing for a different skin colour, despite the positive and self-respecting messages they have been given at home. As we will discuss further in Chap. 3, starting school may be the first time a child encounters the social meaning of their difference from others. It may take the parent or carer by surprise. What may be an innocent question or comment from the child easily becomes freighted with parental fears and a wider political discourse. A simple, matter of fact response which explains and supports self-esteem may be best. The struggle for rights and respect has further to go, despite laws to prevent race, disability and religious discrimination, and the establishment of large ethnic communities through mass migration. The discomfort with people who look different can be maintained by a natural tendency to choose to live with similar others who share values and beliefs.

Think about how you might address this issue if it impacted on your own family, or child. Would you use examples in the lives of people you know, stories, or media, or wait for something relevant to come up? Would you 'go along' with your community values in this case? If not, how would you manage that difference?

Regrettably, traditional attitudes within some migrant groups can also affect the life chances of those with visible difference, where opportunities may be restricted by traditional ideas of social shame. Where possible, connection with advocacy groups in wider society can help these people to live fuller lives if their families permit. These overlapping issues serve to highlight what still needs to change to create shared values and a more inclusive environment, and can be a complex field for the therapist to operate in.

Changing Minds Through Media Visibility: The Pioneers

Though important legislation to protect minorities was first enacted in 1965 this alone was insufficient to create change momentum for other disadvantaged groups. More important is visibility, and pioneering campaigners like Dame Tanni Grey-Thompson, Liz Carr, Davina Ingrams and James Partridge among many others have made a huge difference by stepping into the public eye, challenging the status quo. Twenty years later, between 1982 and 1995, there were 17 attempts to introduce comprehensive and enforceable civil rights for disabled people, before the Disability Discrimination Act was passed into law in 1995, later amended in 2005. This protection includes those with 'severe disfigurements' including scars, birthmarks, diseases of the skin and limb or postural deformation likely to affect their daily life, as well as those with autism and severe mental illness. The campaign to include visible differences in the definition, intended to protect from discrimination, has been controversial for some, as they experience themselves as disabled only by prejudice.

The Shaw Trust's annual list of Britain's 100 most influential disabled people now includes the arts, law, entertainment, business, media and sports sectors, emphasising their commitment to paving the way for others. This list is a very useful resource for therapists working with difference. But for many clients it is still reasonable in a hostile and challenging environment to 'lie low', avoid making demands, or being too visible, although this tends to perpetuate negative assumptions on both sides. The game changers have been those breakthrough individuals in every field who have been able to make connections and cross conceptual barriers, but they are often very talented people who have achieved in an exceptional way despite many obstacles. For someone who has lacked opportunity, support and confidence, the further demand to be outstanding may be experienced as another limitation. Of course, the expectation that they won't be is equally bad! Breaking their own un-necessary limitations is a realistic goal, though this can feel like a huge risk which puts their viability as a human being under scrutiny.

The move from the exception to the norm is a slow process, but there are sometimes breakthrough moments which can be capitalised on. The Channel 4 'Meet the Superhumans' trailer for the 2012 Paralympics, repeated in 2016 as 'We're the Superhumans' which used the Public Enemy song 'Harder than you think' inspired many people. Partly because they looked fierce and amazing, and the production emphasised what they could do, not their limitations. It helped the Paralympics to sell out for the first time, gave Channel 4 its biggest TV audience in 10 years and reportedly changed the way that many people felt about disability. This is the power of the right message, delivered in the right way, at the right time. Though there was some criticism that this perpetuated the prevailing 'exceptionalism' many people found it inspiring and were proud of the team's achievements.

The first Paralympic Games were held in Rome in 1960, and 400 athletes from 23 countries competed, all of whom had spinal cord injuries. Their precursor was held in the UK in 1948, on the opening day of the London Olympics and consisted of 16 men and women archers. It was called the Stoke Mandeville games, conceived as part of their rehabilitation programme. In 1952 Dutch ex-servicemen joined and made it the International Games. They did not have Channel 4 to make their promotion videos, and it took much work behind the scenes to establish the international organisations and funding to support the first full games. There are still some who oppose their inclusion, like Brazilian journalist Joaquim Vieria who called the games in 2016 'a grotesque spectacle' and 'a circus act ... to fill the agenda of political correctness'.

From its very modest beginnings the Paralympics is now a huge multimillion enterprise, but other changes in society have meant that individuals do not have to wait for huge organisations to represent their interests and help their voice to be heard. What they say can be surprising, and via social media people are listening and sharing their messages. That is the good news; the bad is that others have found themselves 'trolled' via the same channels. The media landscape and the arts offer more inclusive programming, and the public are more able to include themselves in the conversation than ever before. In my view, this means that although there may still be broad assumptions which parallel Goffman's disturbing evaluation, there are many more spaces for alternative voices. While there is tremendous pressure for people to conform to stereotyped ideas of physical beauty, there are many others taking on long established discrimination in many areas. One example of this is the very rapid development of the #metoo movement outing sexual abuse in the workplace. This apparently sudden change built on many other smaller groups talking about similar things, and the widespread nature of this shared abuse experience.

Still Some Way to Go Though …

So far the voices of disabled women have been largely absent from the #metoo discourse, although some agencies report they are more likely to experience sexual abuse. Those with visible differences still seem a very long way from being able to achieve something so dramatic, and their pain is not as easily identified with, but changing media representations and awareness of the importance of this are slowly having an impact. One useful examples of the gentle challenge of assumptions is the way that the UK television series 'The Undateables' first created controversy, with doctors and Twitter users describing the title as offensive, playing to the view that disabled and different people were asexual. But after several series since 2012 it has created personalities like Tom who gained 16,000 Twitter followers overnight, and helped others build their careers.

Adam Pearson, a British actor, presenter and campaigner with neurofibromatosis was involved in the production team for the Undateables and 'Beauty and the Beast: the Ugly face of Prejudice' also on Channel 4, but is best known for his 2013 appearance in 'Under the Skin' with Scarlett Johansson. Pearson comments to Elizabeth Day (2014) in an Observer newspaper piece that '*there's a lot of fear around the unknown. If I can try to be as normal as possible and show there's nothing to fear-either on film or day to day, going round the corner to go shopping for milk-then the more people see it in the wider society, the less stigma there is. If I just sit at home and mope, hugging the dog and crying, nothing's going to change.*' But he goes on to point out that facial imperfections are often used as a shorthand for evil in films, whether it be Blofeld's eye scar in James Bond or the villain in Disney's adaptation of the Lone Ranger, whose face was severely scarred and who was given what appeared to be a cleft palate in make-up. '*It's always used very lazily*' explains Pearson. '*In an ideal world, actors with conditions would play characters with these same conditions, but that's a way off. Instead, film makers tend to get a generic, "normal" actor and use prosthetics. If they'd got Adam Sandler and blacked him up to play Nelson Mandela, there would have been an uproar … but with scars and stuff, it seems like people are cool with that.*'

Peter Dinklage is an actor of reduced height who has made a very successful career playing characters of reduced height, so it can be done. He is now widely known now for his performance of Tyrion Lannister in the 'Game of Thrones', and the film 'Three Billboards outside Ebbing, Missouri'. He began acting in 1991 in theatre and made his film debut in 1995 in the independent 'Living in Oblivion' as a bad-tempered dwarf actor, who complains in a dream sequence about stereotyping, '*even I don't have dreams about dwarves!*' (this is a reference to David Lynch's cult TV series Twin Peaks). He has used his roles to explore the experience of being different and the same, challenging assumptions rather than allowing himself to be stereotyped as a comic or sad figure.

Changing the Dominant Narrative: Using Different Media to Communicate Directly

While Dinklage and Pearson's careers have followed a conventional route in some ways, recent years have also seen the emergence of younger vloggers who are able to reach an audience directly on social media without having to seek the approval of 'gatekeepers'. For instance, 13-year-old London based Nikki Lilly has over 2 million YouTube views and 35,000 followers on her site which features make up tutorials, beauty tips and baking alongside sharing her experience of being different. She has AVM, or arteriovenous malformation, a rare condition that is characterised by an abnormal connection between arteries and veins. Nikki now sometimes presents for CBBC, and most notably interviewed then Prime Minister Theresa May, talking about a range of things from Strictly Come Dancing to coping with bullies. The interview was widely praised by the print media, and she later interviewed Jeremy Corbyn, then Opposition leader, not to be outdone. Her positive, honest accounts and relaxed style have been well received. Nikki is unusual as many of the visibly different women who have come to prominence have flawless faces, and while it is now possible to compile a long list of visibly different actors and actresses, very few of these women's faces diverge from the norm.

It can be argued that the first exploration of visible difference in a comic book was the X Men written by Stan Lee and published in 1963. The characters were all mutants with superpowers, living in society but subject to negative prejudice because of their difference. It was a very successful series occurring in parallel with civil rights movements. The first X Men movie was made later in 2000, and emphasised the character's choices about how to deal with their difference and the prejudice they faced, either with anger or with strength and self-assurance. It is notable that the 'bad' mutants are all unhappy about their lot, but the 'goodies' have found a way to accept their true nature. Also, although one way or another all the female characters fail to completely conform to important attractiveness conventions, the male characters are consistently more visually challenging.

However, this too may slowly be changing, as the more recent Spielberg film 'Ready Player One' based on Ernest Cline's book of the same name breaks new ground. It is set in a future world which exaggerates current virtual gaming trends like 'Fortnite'. The characters are all absorbed in an online game called Oasis which is an expansive virtual reality universe. Players adopt personalised avatars to encounter each other in this world, forming rich and intense lives to compensate for the poverty of their real ones. The hero falls in love with the heroine, as usual, and declares his admiration and love for her, after a series of action scenes in which she equals and surpasses him. She then turns him down when he wants to meet in real life, saying he would not like her. Much intense action later they do meet, and it transpires that while both their avatars are exaggerated and idealised versions of themselves, she has an unacknowledged birthmark on her face she is ashamed of. He accepts her anyway (of course) but unlike Beauty and the Beast she is not transformed, instead it gives her the confidence to give her avatar a birthmark as well. They win the day together, matching each other in courage and energy.

It may seem a minor thing, but as young people become more engrossed in virtual game worlds and social media it does open up some interesting questions about how people construct their identities, what is considered real and what is not, and how this might change in the future opening up a useful space for therapy. Already researchers are looking at possible uses of avatars in online type platforms to help teach autistic children how to interact socially. (Hopkins et al. 2011)

What Media Do Your Clients Relate to?

This is all very interesting, but what does it mean for the therapist and their client? I would argue that (more than ever) it is of utmost importance to understand the client's personal points of reference in film TV, books and other media, and how these impact on their sense of who they are. This will be very different for someone who grew up in the 1960s and 1970s, compared with the 1990s and 2000s. Discussion of these narratives can inform treatment and develop a shared understanding about how their sense of self has been constructed, and how they might want to change. Role models in the media, both trying, making mistakes, and succeeding, can create a field of meaning and possibility for the individual which helps them find the courage to experiment in their own way.

Festinger's Social Comparison Theory (1954) first used the term 'social comparison' to propose the idea that a drive exists in people to evaluate their opinions and abilities in comparison with others. He drew on earlier studies of social groups, group dynamics, social communication and conformity to evidence his ideas and argued that people would first seek an objective benchmark, but when these were not available, they would compare themselves with those around them, using 'upward' or 'downward' comparisons. For instance, a writer might compare themselves with a successful more experienced writer (upward), or a much less experienced one (downward). He regarded the judgements that were made as generally reliable when people compared themselves with others like them. In other words, this social 'norming' can create shared assumptions and cohesion. If no others 'like them' are readily available, or there is a habitual bias in one direction, it is easy to see how problems can be amplified.

So, for clients with a visible difference there can be complications in comparison. Who are your clients' most frequent references? Do you have access to how they manage their internal narratives around this issue?

Since this early work researchers have studied the changes brought by the growing influence of mass media, compared with more intimate sources such as friends and family (Irving 1990). Others have also found that comparison on the dimension of physical appearance tends to be upwards (to those perceived as better looking), rather than downwards, creating decrements in perception (Wheeler and Miyake 1992). Self-discrepancy theory and self-schema theory are both cognitive processing models which suggest the way a person internally represents themselves determines how they respond to media messages, noting individual differences in the way appearance schemas and self-discrepancies are held. This accounts for differences in vulnerability to media messages (Altabe and Thompson 1996; Dittmar and Halliwell 2008). Analysis directs the therapist towards opportunities for constructive change, though the categories of 'up and down' are not always useful.

Katy's Story

Of course, how someone sees themselves is determined by the messages they receive from their environment, though this is not a passive process. Katy, a 20-year-old biology student, had a supportive family and some great friends. Her studies were going well. The problem that brought her into therapy was that she had never had a close relationship, something she longed for, and she believed this was because she was less attractive than all her friends.

In her first session she said 'nobody wants to get involved with me once they discover I only have one leg. It's too complicated. They just don't want the hassle.' Her social media was full of photos of her looking great, at parties with friends, very much part of her milieu it seemed, and she was happy to share this. So her therapist took some time to wonder with her, trying to understand how she was explaining the problem to herself. Her lower left leg had been amputated as a result of a family car crash when she was 9 years old.

(continued)

(continued)

Before then she had been a sporty girl, like her brothers. Her physical recovery had gone well and her school friends were very supportive, but she could no longer take part in the team sports she enjoyed. Her friends were entering a stage when they as a group were becoming more interested in style, clothes and following people they liked on social media, so it wasn't a big problem. Her parents had suggested that she join 'a sports team for people with disabilities', but she found she had little in common with them, saying 'it just felt like a random group of people'. Sports stopped being part of her life.

Katy was a lovely young woman, doing her best to deal with the regular challenges of life at her age. She had a couple of close friends, who she talked to when she was let down once again by someone she met on a dating site and really liked, who ghosted her after a couple of dates. Two weeks later she learned (via social media) that he was seeing another person in her group. They said things like 'well, he's just really immature like that' and 'you're too good for him'. Which didn't help. Checking her rival's profile, she found it hard to understand, apart from the leg thing, as she said, breaking down in tears. 'I feel that whatever I do people will always see me as inferior. I can't solve this.' She began withdrawing from people, something that really concerned her close friends.

Her therapist, using a values-based approach, spent a few sessions with Katy exploring the things that really mattered to her, a process she found interesting, realising she had been waylaid by her recent disappointments. Of course one of them was a good, close relationship, and this led easily to a discussion of the qualities she wanted in a partner. They made a list with this on one side. On the other side they reflected together on what such a person might be looking for in their partner. This was more painful, connecting with the grief, shame and fear that had brought her to therapy which her therapist responded to empathically. During this process they agreed that although the crash and amputation had been handled well enough at the time, it was helpful to explore the ongoing impact on her feelings about herself. It was also an opportunity to help her acknowledge all the really great things about who she was, while accepting at that moment she did not feel they were enough.

Returning to her use of social media, her therapist suggested that she might look at the profiles of some celebrities and athletes with 'visible differences' between sessions, and next time they talked about who she liked and didn't, and differences in the way they presented themselves. She started following a couple. Returning to her 'ideal partner' checklist, they talked more about what special qualities that person might need (if any) to be her partner. Would they need to understand what she had been through? How and when might she communicate this? Was it OK for them to say it

(continued)

(continued)

was too much for them to deal with? If they did, what did that mean about her? Something/nothing/it depends? These are very difficult questions, and Katy opted to explore online what other young people in similar situations were saying. Of course she kept in touch with her old friends too and found after a while that she felt comfortable letting them know more about what she was going through. Learning how to talk about difference, and feel OK with herself doing that was part of her recovery process.

(NOTE: this is a very short summary of part of therapeutic work)

More recent research shows that a bias towards 'downward comparison' among those with visible differences is associated with greater resilience. The correction of unhelpful cognitive bias is one measure of the usefulness of a therapy episode, as these left unresolved will create further problems. Although to achieve positive change discrimination needs to be addressed within the individuals concerned, and this is the focus for individual therapy, change is also powerfully created by those who can resist the accepted stereotypes and assert different narratives of self in a social context. Breaking the pattern of withdrawal and self-exclusion is an agent for change both within the individual and the wider group, as a way of undermining long held and restricting beliefs, creating a virtuous cycle.

For instance, in the same way that social skills training is an effective method to support individuals experiencing appearance related distress, it can also facilitate greater understanding if offered to whole classes at school. This can build recognition that these skills are needed by all to understand a variety of differences and improve social relations. In this way children and young people can learn early and easily the way that uses of language can construct difference or facilitate understanding and acceptance. We will explore further the possibilities for influencing the school and social environment in the chapters on family and development.

References

Altabe MN, Thompson JK (1996) Body image: a cognitive self-schema construct? Cognitive Therapy Research 20:171–193

Barker P (2012) Toby's Room Penguin.

Bateson G (2002) Mind and nature: a necessary unity. Hampton Press Inc.

Brune JA, Wilson DJ (2013) Disability and passing. Temple University Press, Philadelphia

Dittmar H, Halliwell E (2008) Think 'ideal' and feel bad? Using self-discrepancies to understand negative media effects. In: Dittmar H (ed) Consumer culture identity and wellbeing: the search for the 'good life and the 'body perfect'. Psychology Press, Hove

Elizabeth Day (2014) How Scarlett Johannsen helped me challenge disfigurement stigma. In: The Observer, Film Sunday 13th April 2014

Falvey H (2012) Cross cultural differences. In: Rumsey N, Harcourt D (eds) The Oxford handbook of the psychology of appearance. Oxford University Press

Festinger (1954) A theory of social comparison processes. Hum Relat 7(2):117–140. Sage Journals

Gergen K J (1985) The social constructionist movement in modern psychology. Am Psychol 40(3):266–275

Goffman E (1963) Stigma: notes on the management of spoiled identity. Penguin Books

Hopkins IM, Gower M, Perez TA, Biasini F (2011) *Journal of Autism and Developmental Disorders* 41(11):1543–1555

Irving LM (1990) Mirror Images: effects of the standard of beauty on the self and body esteem of women exhibiting varying levels of bulimic symptoms. *Journal of Social and Clinical Psychology* 9(2):230–242

Longmore P (2003) Screening stereotypes, images of disabled people in television and motion pictures. In: Why I burned my book, and other essays on disability. Temple University Press, Philadelphia

Nelson JA (1994) The disabled, the media, and the information age. Greenwood Publishing Group, pp 1–24

Orbach S (2009) Bodies. Profile Books, London

O'Toole JM (2003) 'Passing for White'. University of Massachusetts Press.

Shaffer DR, Crepaz N, Sun CR, (2000) Physical attractiveness stereotyping in cross cultural perspective: similarities and differences between Americans and Taiwanese. *Journal of Cross-Cultural Psychology* 31(5):557–582

Tuchman G, (1979) Women's depiction by the mass media, in signs. *Journal of Women in Culture and Society* 3:528–542

Wheeler and Miyake (1992) Social comparison in everyday life. *Journal of Personality and Social Psychology* 62(5):760–773

Widdows H (2018) Perfect me: beauty as an ethical ideal. Oxford and Princeton University Press

Wilensky AS (2000) 'Passing for Normal'. Broadway Books.

Wood JT, (1994) Gendered Lives Commun Gend Cult, Chapter 9. Wadsworth Belmont California, pp 231–244

3

The Developing Self: The Differences of Difference

As all psychology students know, the development of selfhood occurs as the child discovers who they are over time through interaction with others. Their 'personhood' is shaped in communication firstly with the primary carer, family group and later the community. From the earliest days the baby is gathering experiences that over time will inform them of who others think they are. By touching their own face and body and those of others they begin to experience their influence on the world, and the difference between themselves and other people. Developmental theorists differ in emphasising the significance of the individual and social context. But understanding of the self, created through interaction with others, is a lifelong process as we grow and age.

The First Adjustments to Difference

In Western societies the early social environment is seen primarily as the responsibility of the parent or carer if they are capable. Caring for a newborn is a significant adjustment for any new parent. But those who must also quickly adapt to caring for a different child have a series of extra

© The Author(s) 2020
V. Purcell, *Understanding Visible Differences*, Palgrave Texts in Counselling and Psychotherapy, https://doi.org/10.1007/978-3-030-51655-0_3

challenges, both practical and emotional. As antenatal support improves many mothers will now have been advised that their child has problems prior to the birth, during a routine scan. A facial cleft occurs at 5–11 weeks of gestation, and in the UK this can now be detected during an ultrasound scan at 20 weeks. Spina Bifida occurs in the first four weeks of pregnancy, so can also be detected during ultrasound, if not at a 16-week amniocentesis test, unless it is a very mild form. A maternal blood test can detect 95–99% of foetal chromosomal abnormalities at 9–10 weeks of pregnancy, but these are expensive and not routinely given in the UK at this time.

At this point the mother may be asked to make an informed decision if there is a problem. There is very little time for this momentous choice, and parents report feeling under pressure, struggling to work through the ramifications of continuing with the pregnancy for themselves and their child. Accurate and timely diagnosis, with quick link to information and specialist help is important, though not all possible outcomes are clear at this early stage. Brown (2012) found that the way the news is given, the quality and accuracy of information, and the support given are significant factors in parental adjustment. She goes on to comment that if this is well managed it tends to result in a better birthing experience. Pregnancy can be terminated at 21 weeks in case of severe foetal handicap, but current professional opinion is that in this case it is best if the baby is born dead. If the parents agree to the procedure their baby is killed by injection prior to the birth. This is an awful, traumatic experience for the parents, who may feel isolated and guilty for making this choice, even though it has been supported by health professionals.

> If your client needed help or support with issues related to this would you know how to advise them? If not, where would you look for assistance?

For others, who have embroidered their dreams of who their baby is and will be during pregnancy, the birth experience will include the shock and fear of discovery that they are different, and initial reactions may be of disgust and horror. It helps if the nursing staff have been trained to react in an understanding and supportive way, which parents report lessens their distress, but even experienced staff may lack information and support in working with unusual babies. Adult interviewees give accounts of nurses bursting into tears, or the baby being rushed away, leaving them to imagine the worst. The new parent(s) may need to abandon their initial expectations and grieve the loss of the wished-for baby at least in the short term, though hope and encouragement can mean a lot. One new mother commented on the support of the nurse specialist after the birth, recalling how important it was to her when the nurse said 'don't give up on your dreams'. Another, older, interviewee said '*when I was born the nurses asked my mother if I was to be given away, upon which she exclaimed "of course not, she's beautiful". So I became the first facially deformed baby born in that exclusive Georgetown hospital to be kept by the parents (as generally they were given away for adoption).*' For the person concerned this family re-telling is a precious story of being truly wanted, but often the circumstances of their birth are not discussed, or not in a helpful way. Being told by an aunt that 'I just burst into tears when I first saw you' is not a confidence-builder.

Discovering What Is Involved

Following the birth another accommodation may be needed to a period of medical interventions and tests, depending on the condition. A Swedish study by Johanssen and Ringsberg (2004) found that parents reported trauma after the discovery of a cleft, but slowly adjusted, and they report that stage models of grieving which identify periods of shock, disbelief and anger can be helpful to parents trying to understand and manage their own emotional responses. The mental health of the parent prior to the birth, family and systemic factors also need to be considered in supporting the adjustment process. For parents who have made an active choice to continue with the pregnancy, there can be times of anxiety and remorse as their newborn baby undergoes painful procedures, guilt for making a choice which causes their child so much distress, and fears about future stigma they and their baby will experience.

There is rarely a context to discuss the impact of these experiences on everyone concerned, which may be relevant for your client when reflecting on their own memories.

Researchers have investigated the impact of this shock on attachment strength and styles in craniofacial conditions, which might be thought to impact most severely on attachment, as eye contact is so important to this and synchrony. Early studies seemed to indicate that mothers showed reduced eye contact, play and smiling with facially different babies (Field and Vega-Lahr 1984), but this has not been supported by later researchers. Among others Leong et al. (2017) found few differences between these children and the control group. Maris et al. (2000) and Coy et al. (2002) found more secure attachments, which they interpreted as due to the increased protectiveness of the mother. Generally, researchers in earlier papers have tended to focus on deficits, which may be understandable in a period when minority voices were rarely included in the design of research.

The preference for attractive over unattractive white female faces in 2–3-day-old infants was first noted by Slater (2000), which invites the thought that this preference might be innate. Later researchers found that this was not the case, as experiments with even younger babies failed to find it. It seems that the preference develops at a very early stage, and a possible explanation is offered by Hoss and Langlois (2003) who suggest that the early infant 'averages' across familiar faces they have seen. Evidence for this early preference is supported by other researchers, though there is no research to date on the impact of having a visually different carer on this preference. Hoss and Langlois also found that 6-month-old babies showed an attractiveness bias when looking at white male, black female and infant faces, though the bias is most pronounced in female faces. The absence of visibly different faces in books, media and public life, which has been noted by media researchers, will tend to perpetuate this bias if the 'averaging' hypothesis is correct. However in interview, parents with visible differences say that their children, and their friends, have never commented on their appearance, accepting it as a family norm though they were prepared for a 'talk'. Separately, the children also say it was never an issue for them, perhaps indicating that in loving close relationships the bias is not relevant.

The child does not develop what is generally understood as a sense of self until about 2 years of age, when they are able to recognize themselves in a mirror or photo, though earlier than this they may be able to make self-statements like 'I am a good boy/girl'. The distinctions between I, me, you and mine arrive with language skills, and by 3 years the child will demonstrate emotions which relate to the self, like embarrassment, pride, guilt and shame.

'Beauty Is Good'

Dion (1973) first found that the stereotype 'beauty is good' emerges at about 3 years of age, by which time children show a preference for attractive playmates. This bias is associated with friendliness and laughter, while unattractive faces are associated with crying and negative tones. Following on from this Ramsay and Langlois (2002) found that five-year-old children had better memory for beautiful female characters in stories that were consistent with the 'beauty is good' stereotype (for instance Beauty and the Beast, Snow White etc.), though this bias was not found with male characters. Once again there is no research on whether this bias is also present in children of visibly different parents.

It appears that a preference established very early is then elaborated on, absorbing reinforcing narratives from the family environment and culture. In a market economy this is likely to be magnified, as there is little profit in contradicting it, and it is worth noting that a narrow definition of beauty undermines the confidence of children from minority cultures as well as those who are 'average' if they are not represented. Smolak (2010, 2012) reports that in an analysis of books and videos aimed at 4–8 year-olds 72% showed an association between beauty and being loved, and of course this representation of beauty is unlikely to be ethnically inclusive. This is changing, but it highlights the importance of selecting the stories and images a child is exposed to. Body shape concerns also emerge by about 3 years old, with children viewing overweight peers as having more negative characteristics. With the rise of social media, and marketing aimed directly at younger children, awareness of the risk to healthy self-esteem in children is rising.

The new parent of a different child, particularly one with facial difference, must consciously work at establishing their child's self-confidence and maintaining it through childhood, when there will be many challenges. The messages that the child receives at home about what makes a good and attractive person are important. Living with a congenital condition is likely to impact on self-perceptions, with the risk that the child internalizes the negative views of some of their peers and makes attributions to the self from difficult interpersonal experiences. This can lead to poorer emotional adjustment and cognitive functioning. Here is a comment, looking back

> *I wish I had known in my childhood that my mother had said I was beautiful. My difference was never referred to (out of mistaken tact), so it became my private curse. I asked God daily what I had done to deserve such a curse, and why couldn't I be beautiful like my sisters (they made the same prayer though I didn't know it then). I nursed the vain hope that one day I would turn into a beautiful princess. Then the moment came when I realized I would have the same face all my life—I was horrified!*
>
> *Whenever I had to look in the mirror, say to brush my hair, I would make the centre of my face go blurry, so I didn't really know what I looked like, I had lost my face! When, at 15 a kindly plastic surgeon asked me what I would like done about it, all I could do was let tears roll down my face. I had been a sad child, though showing a brave front. I do wonder at what point I lost my laughter.*

This is a difficult subject to broach, unless your client brings it up. How might you go about it, if you thought it was relevant? Even if it remains unspoken, how might these early messages be influencing your client's current issues?

Learning How to Deal with Prejudice

To thrive, different children need to be able to understand and cope with the occasional staring, blunt questions and anxieties of others, and feel good about themselves and their bodies. This requires a higher level of social competence than their peers may have. This may sound like an almost impossible task under duress, but it can be achieved. Eugene Grant, a writer and charity trustee from Newcastle has recently described his experiences of street abuse on the way to work and in pubs for BBC News (31st August 2018). Despite his difficult experiences with negative unwanted attention he has developed assertive coping skills to deal with it and says '*some days it doesn't bother me at all and I just get on with it, … and some days it really upsets me. … It can chip away a bit, but he also comments "I love being a dwarf person, I love my body, I love my community".* Through the Restricted Growth Association he uses his own experiences to support young people around the country, and call out thoughtless behaviour. A developing child needs opportunity to understand and cope with negative experiences in ways that are congruent with their stage of development, and stories, images and real-life mentors all help to create an alternative narrative.

> What coping skills does your client use most often, and why do they favour those?

The work of building a positive and resilient self-image ideally also requires the help of an understanding support network, which may be the wider family or other groups with experience to offer. There is little academic research focusing on the messages families give to their children which are not weight-related. A few studies report that families which give positive messages about appearance tended to have children with more positive body image (Bearman et al. 2006) though the content of these messages matters. When they concern things that are within the child's control, and easily changeable, like hairstyle, clothes and behaviours, this is associated with confidence (Frisen and Holmqvist 2010). What is communicated needs to be consistent with implicit family values, and congruent with other experiences. Most importantly the locus of the problem should be clearly identified as outside of the child. Other people's attitudes are their responsibility. One interviewee commented 'my mum is my protection barrier' and told of occasions when her mother had asked other parents in public places to please stop their children from staring, offering to explain if they have a question. She found this very helpful and has grown into a confident young woman.

> What stories does your client have about how other people around them have helped them to deal with similar situations?

Parents need to find good answers to their child's questions when they experience negative reactions and staring, ones which protect their self-esteem and build resilience and social skill. If a parent tells their child they are beautiful to them, explaining in what way matters, as does being realistically positive. It can help to explain that some people are thoughtless, uninformed or prejudiced, and their comments should not be internalized. (It's their problem!) The everyday processing of ideas and images in the family context is also important; otherwise the child will come to feel that their loving parent doesn't understand their experiences in the wider social world, or worse, does not really mean what they say.

This can be hard work! A support group with parenting experience related to visible difference can provide much needed help and encouragement which is difficult for health professionals to replicate, and the immediacy of online resources has made this much more accessible in recent years. It is hoped that parents will have been informed of these resources as part of a support package offered postnatally. If not, support groups for specific issues have a wealth of experience to share.

Diana Baumrind (1991) comments on the influence of parenting style on the development of their child's self-concept and coping skills. A parent who is securely attached themselves and not overprotective, with an authoritative (not authoritarian) parenting style is most easily able to encourage a positive attitude to new experience, and resilience in the face of difficulty. However, the value of these characteristics has been found to vary cross-culturally, with other researchers noting that a demanding, authoritarian style produced culturally valued outcomes in education. Positive self-esteem and self-autonomy were not associated with good school performance in the UAE (Alsheikh et al. 2015).

Self-esteem and Coping in Social Situations

Young children aged from 2–4 show an increase in social behaviour once they have established a self-concept. Playgroups provide an opportunity for wider interaction under parental supervision. As they develop interaction alters, from 'parallel play' to more confident exchanges, and real friendships based on shared play and interests are formed. By this time most children are attending school, and teacher attitudes and knowledge are critical. Sadly, some teachers will also be influenced by the same 'beauty is good' bias, and accounts of bullying at school given in Lansdown et al. (1997) of those with congenital disfigurement make sad reading. Strikingly though, as one contributor comments 'even at that date I knew about "facial discrimination"'. I said to the teacher (in response to an investigation for misbehaviour) 'You only asked Deborah and me again because we are the two ugliest girls in the class, and it's not me!' (Katherine Lacy, then in her 50s, p. 22, Lansdown et al. 1997). Somewhere this woman had developed the confidence to speak up even in a situation where she might have felt powerless, and at a time when prejudice was less likely to be challenged. This is a striking testament to supportive relationships in other areas of her life, though it is worth noting that the influence of television and social media would have been much less as she grew up.

> Parents who are concerned about their child's transition to school can assist their child by offering the teacher and school resources to help them understand their child's needs, and several charities give access to these (see Appendix).

What Does Developmental Theory and Research Say?

As you would expect, quite a lot, which I will not summarise here. It is worth reminding yourself of factors which influence self-esteem. Argyle (2008) identified four—(1) the reaction of others, as we have noted potentially more complicated for a child who looks different. He comments that if loving others admire, flatter, seek us out and attend to what we say this contributes to the development of a positive self-image. A visibly different child is less likely to be admired physically, so competence in a domain which is respected is very important.

> What do you know about how your client processes meaning in this area. What strategies do they use to protect their self-esteem?

(2) Comparison with others is something that everyone does. If the people we compare ourselves to appear 'better' than us in domains that matter, there is a risk of poor self-image, this was Katy's issue. For this reason, having contact with peers who also differ from the 'normal' is helpful as the young adult or child's sense of who they are socially develops. (3) Social roles matter, and for a younger child this also means who their family are in society. If their family group are successful and respected by others this can contribute to a positive feeling, alternatively a stigmatized family identity will have the opposite effect. This does not have to be material success; community respect is an achievable equivalent. (4) Finally, the extent to which an individual identifies with others matters— they need to feel part of the group, with important and valued factors in common. Cultural factors are also important here, and how much importance the community places on 'we' rather than 'I'.

Argyle found that the relationship between the 'ideal self', that is who someone thinks they should be, and the person they think they are is likely to affect how much they value themselves, and their measured self-esteem throughout life. The wider the gulf between these two, the lower self-esteem will be, a clear focus for therapeutic work on values and self-image. Reflecting on this, Eugene Grant's assertive appreciation of his body and his community is significant, and it is clearly important (to him) to state that he values his appearance, to counter the pitying assumption that everyone would prefer to be 'normal'. In fact, most people with a visible difference would choose to have the same chances in life and not be discriminated against or bullied. When asked, most do not say they would prefer to look like someone else, though as interest in cosmetic enhancement becomes mainstream more older adults with visible differences seek improvements on their earlier surgery.

> Would you choose to look like someone else? If your private answer is yes, what difference do you think it would make? If it is no, what does that mean about you?

Developmental theorists have disagreed about whether development is continuous, involving gradual and ongoing changes throughout the lifespan, or whether it is staged, with each stage building on the competencies of the previous ones. These two are not necessarily exclusive-development could be discontinuous and staged, according to the demands and opportunities in front of the person, and the resources available to them. In therapy creating a space with greater potential can facilitate new growth. Stage models of the development of self provide a helpful way to consider the developmental and social requirements of each stage of life, even though they may not be as linear and clear cut as some theories propose. Four of the most notable are those of Erikson, Piaget, Marcia (2012) and Vygotsky, though later developmental researchers have added much important and qualifying material. The primarily Western idea of the 'self' and the social project of creating autonomous adults assumed by these theories has also been challenged as culturally specific, which has required contemporary therapists to more carefully consider the context and aspirations of their clients, and their own assumptions. This can be a complex area however, as the child also has rights, even if they are not fully recognized in the family, or wider society.

Can you think of something in your own life that you did not learn at the expected 'stage', but acquired later? For some this might be a skill, like swimming, for others understanding a social 'rule' was specific to a particular time or place. Or something about yourself.

More contemporary theorists have elaborated these simple staged models in ways that help us understand the more complex situations of modern life. The pressures, hierarchies and multiple voices created by migration and mass media, including social media are mapped more carefully. Intersectionality, a term attributed to Professor Kimberley Crenshaw (1991), attempts to capture the way that different types of discrimination intersect in multiple and simultaneous ways, creating a unique experience of discrimination which is not summative. Nash (2008) uses an identity theory to also consider the agency that different aspects of identity permit in different contexts. Both are presented in Butler (2015) who describes how she uses these ideas in therapy training, with the same scenario discussed in small groups in relation to people with a different age/gender/ethnicity/disability. She found that trainees were more comfortable focusing on their 'own' areas, anxious and sometimes over-cautious when dealing with difference. This is a useful thought experiment for practising therapists, to check their own areas of discomfort.

> Having an area of 'discomfort' is pretty normal it seems. Have you had the experience of coming across one in a therapy session? It could be when your client reveals views you strongly disagree with in some way for instance. What did you do, and how might you improve on that next time?

John Burnham (2012) and colleagues developed the acronym 'social graces' to represent aspects of difference in beliefs, power and lifestyle, visible and invisible, voiced and unvoiced, which should be considered in the therapy relationship. Since then the category has grown and currently includes: gender, geography, race, religion, age, ability, appearance, class, culture, ethnicity, education, employment, sexuality, sexual orientation and spirituality. This means the acronym is now GGRRAAAACCEEESSS. Alongside this is a greater recognition of multiple aspects of self, and the 'process' nature of identity, an ongoing social, internal and interpersonal dialogue through life which the therapist steps into for a period. Development continues as an adult, potentially into old age, and though this was first noted by Erikson the extended time now spent as an older adult is a new field of exploration.

Is Acquired Difference Different?

This chapter begins with a look at those born with congenital differences, but we will now consider the experiences of those who have had a relatively normal start to life, with all the experiences and assumptions about the self that this involves. A crisis which causes traumatic change to physical appearance, whether through accident or illness may throw everything the person has believed about themselves into question. The age at which this happens is significant, as they will have only the psychological resources available at their stage of development, as my brief description of Katy's therapy indicates. This knowledge of self, and its traumatic change, is in contrast to the unfolding complexity of growing up 'different' in the eyes of others, coming to understand what that means, coping with multiple challenges to the development of healthy self-esteem, and hopefully many opportunities to build resilience over time.

Protecting a Good Relationship with Ourselves

In our media saturated society, only a very small minority of men and women have faces and bodies similar to those idealized in the media. Most of us are less likely to win the real-time beauty contest, and the popularity of 'beauty face' apps to improve social media images demonstrates a wide concern about being 'good enough'. The pervasiveness of these images has led sociocultural theorists to argue that continued exposure leads to an observer perspective on the self. Children often have an acute sense of what and who is 'normal', and what is not, and what they 'should' be like. Social pressures on appearance are apparent from the early school years. Lowes and Tiggemann (2003) found in their UK study of dieting awareness and body shape that 59% of 5–8-year-old girls wanted to be thinner, and only 24% were satisfied with their body size! In the same study 30% of boys were satisfied, 35% wanted to be bigger, and 35% thinner. By their teens both girls and boys spend a substantial amount of their own money on clothes, and a growing minority are supported by parents in their wish to have cosmetic surgery. This seemingly relentless pressure for a more enhanced appearance, often defined in a very narrow way, is in contradiction to the increased awareness and respect for the rights of different others, and the visibility of difference. At this time we can only speculate about the likely outcome, but each brave person who speaks out can more easily find like-minded others in the internet age.

Do you have a specific pose or expression you frequently adopt for photos? This was spoofed in 'Upstart Crow' on TV as a 'selfington portraiture', to hilarious effect (season 2, episode 7, 2016). But what do you think it means about how we think of ourselves?

Frederickson and Roberts (1997) offer their self-objectification theory to explain the process which leads people to believe that their motivation to improve their appearance is a free choice. The body becomes valued more for how it looks than what it can accomplish. Their research was initially conducted with women, but later found to also apply to men in certain aspects of appearance. Weilage and Hope (1999) note that once looks are objectified people are more vulnerable to feedback which implies that they do not meet societal standards.

While very young children do not typically engage in much social comparison, from primary school age to adolescence they do so increasingly. Access to computer technology, Instagram, Snapchat and YouTube are common, reinforcing beliefs about attractiveness and beauty which become components of self-evaluation concerning appearance. Where a physical trauma occurs in later childhood or adulthood their established beliefs about themselves may be threatened or destroyed. For this reason, access to mirrors is often restricted in trauma departments and the process of becoming acquainted with their changed appearance is managed, alongside the provision of psychological support if needed.

James Partridge was seriously burned on the face and body at the age of 18 during a car crash, and he writes movingly of his treatment and path to recovery as well as his appreciation of the medical staff. He says *'Many facial injuries result from split-second tragedies that throw their victims out of their habitual lifestyle and into an alien world of hospitals, medicine and highly technical life-saving skills and equipment'*. He goes on to describe the very lengthy treatment process, and what he discovered along the way about his changed face and life.

> *What you have lost in being disfigured are two social advantages. First, you have lost the chance of being automatically accepted into any social gathering as just an ordinary person. You will always be noticeable and will feel continually "on trial". … Secondly, your facial damage brings you much unwanted attention. You stick out in crowds, you are noticeable wherever you go. If you fail to give convincing answers in this public inquisition, you fear that people will interpret this as further evidence that your facial disfigurement conceals a low-value personality.* (Partridge 1990)

Trauma and Recovery

This is James' personal account of his journey, and as an articulate and well-resourced person with supportive family and friends he had many advantages in his crisis. But over time his frank description has struck a chord with, and he has helped, many people through the charity he established. This transition from someone who had a right to privacy and acceptance, to someone who is always different is stark and well described. The person living through it must mourn not just the loss of the public self so far created, but an imagined future self and life. This is a psychological crisis, but also an opportunity for change and post traumatic growth with the right support. Recognition and treatment of psychological trauma in these circumstances is more frequently offered by specialist hospital departments.

> For the patient, discharge is just the beginning of a different life, and the moment of change may need to be revisited more than once, at different life stages.

Outcomes for patients with serious burns vary in a complex way, but PTSD associated with the injury is also associated with poorer functional outcomes and adjustment post-injury (Corry et al. 2010). It is recognized that although anyone can suffer a traumatic accident of this type, burns patients are more likely to have pre-existing psychopathology than the general population. A small number will have burned themselves intentionally while in psychological distress. Conversely, both random and targeted attacks involving acid are increasing in large cities. Helpful coping styles, like positive self-talk rather than avoidance is associated with a good recovery, as are good interactional skills. Having a range of skills which are flexibly deployed seems to be a significant factor (Robinson 1997).

The recovery process is lengthy, and for adolescents and young adults peer support is very important. Burn Camps for younger children have very positive qualitative reviews and aim to encourage the children to test their boundaries and gain confidence in the company of professionals, like play specialists, psychologists, volunteers and other survivors. Though organised support groups are not for everyone, the chance to network and learn from peers can be invaluable. Katie Piper, who was attacked as a young woman with acid by a confederate of her ex-boyfriend, comments on the importance of being with similar others (describing treatment in France) *'and then you go to this scar management centre. I was wearing a plastic mask, there were other people in the classes wearing the mask, I was going to the pool and seeing other people's bodies that were scarred and I wasn't thrown back into society, I was around similar people. … I could see one woman who had been there and come back a year on and she'd been wearing the mask and it motivated me to keep wearing it because I could see her results. The morale was good between patients, you could laugh and joke with people. You didn't feel that you didn't fit in, you didn't have those feelings of not being worthy'* (from Cadogan 2010).

She goes on to describe a lengthy and difficult process of recovery, good days and bad, and the importance of a supportive family and friends. Katie has gone on to establish her own foundation to help others, and to appear in TV programmes like 'My Beautiful Friends' to increase public understanding, as well as a competing in Strictly Come Dancing 2018.

Becoming Independent

By adolescence the differing expectations and experiences of young men and women become more marked, and this is the moment when the potential negative impact of visible difference on the person's romantic opportunities, future career success and possible happiness are more likely to be felt. Bourdieu's (1986) description of the body as social capital—either bringing entitled access to social resources, free of prejudicial treatment, or depriving others of access and exposing them to maltreatment becomes more salient. It may also be the time when the limitations of medical interventions and plastic surgery become clearer (if they have had multiple surgeries while developing), and they truly understand they will always be different from others. Others are still waiting for cosmetic improvements, and delays are felt keenly. One young woman described her devastation after her rhinoplasty was postponed before she went to university. Another said that she had hers 2 days before the start of college, meaning that she had to travel in for her registration with all her dressings still in place. Having someone with her helped to manage the staring, and she underwent a further 2 operations during her course. To cope, a group of supportive and trusted friends are often relied on, and more wide-ranging encounters avoided, sometimes limiting opportunities in a new environment.

> Can you think of someone from your own clinical practice (who does not have a visible difference) fitting this description? How would their treatment have been complicated if they had looked different?

This can be a very complex stage, when anxieties are unmediated by positive adult experiences, and the 'scaffolding' offered by parents, educators and society in general towards a settled adult life may seem inadequate to the challenge. Particularly in the post-school student/trainee stage a lack of structure, combined with separation from previous supportive social networks can lead to an anxious and defensive avoidance of study and people. Psychoanalytic theorists like Erikson (1980) consider this stage as a second individuation process, commenting on the importance of the mentoring function in correcting 'old scripts' and overcoming identity confusion in a creative and life-enhancing way. Unfortunately, in contemporary further education the opportunities to develop these helpful relationships with mentors are rare. Where support services exist, they are under tremendous pressure, and few can offer the chance to form a connection with a counsellor or psychologist for brief work and ongoing follow-up contact when needed. Researchers working in this area note that although the adolescent transition provides possibly the greatest opportunity for positive change (something which usually happens over time and may require periodic support), it is also very difficult to engage this age group in treatment. It may be at this stage they feel least likely to be understood without judgement, and their important challenges of success socially and in accomplishment do not immediately seem advanced by engaging in a therapeutic relationship with someone much older. A more peer focused approach has the advantage of offering important social engagement and avenues for connection, but can put additional strain on those offering support at a time when they have their own challenges.

> If you were designing an environment to facilitate the process of transition from adolescent to young adult what would it look like? Would it resemble university in some/any ways? What advantages or disadvantages are there to making it shorter or longer (excluding operational ones)? How many years is the 'right' amount of time to spend on it?

Gender and Difference

Although the pressures on young women and men are likely to be gendered, bringing into focus potential issues for those working out their sexual identity, there is more current research on visible differences in this age group which either aims to be gender-neutral or focuses on the pressures and difficulties young women experience. Some of this work provides interesting points of reference and contrast when exploring the experiences of men, but the lion's share of research funding is allocated to weight related disorders.

As one example Piran's Developmental Theory of Embodiment (2017) examines the 'body journeys' of a diverse group of young women through early childhood to adolescence and later years. From a radical feminist position, it explores the salience of the body to people's identities, adopting perspectives from Erikson (1985) and Merlau-Ponty in Iawakuma (2002) to explore individual perceptions of how their bodies matter to their identity. This is a potentially restorative view, offering a framework for change when someone may have been damaged by negative messages from their culture, and contrasts positive body image, deconstructed into different domains with negative body image. For instance, the 'Mental Domain' in positive body image includes mental freedom and a critical stance towards social discourses, which creates the space for freedom of choice in many areas. Its (negative) opposite has mental 'corseting' instead of freedom, through accepting the idea of the body and by extension the self as deficient in object-related social discourses. This in turn disrupts body connection and comfort, restricts agency, and interferes with the person's connection to desire. Instead of attuned self-care, there is disrupted attunement, self-harm and neglect, with the body inhabited as an objectified site. The seeming ascendancy of this perspective is seen in an increase in steroid use in men to develop their muscles in conjunction with exercise, and TV viewing which is focused on the body as a means of 'winning', such as 'Love Island' and 'Naked Attraction'.

> As people age they often become less identified with their physical appearance. After all, they used to look different. In what ways is this similar to the attitude of someone with a visible difference who has undergone surgery which changes their appearance? In what ways is it different in your view?

Piran (2017) argues that it does not make sense to tell anyone to feel good about their bodies without providing them with actual positive experiences of being embodied which develop a sense of wellbeing. This experiential approach also offers examples of ways that adult women can recapture physical and mental freedom and move from disempowerment and disconnection to experiencing themselves as having social power. This perspective does not consider the experience of people whose physical self is transformed through illness, accident or surgery, or those 'born different' who may undergo transformations through surgery. Their relationship with their bodily identity will be different, through the experience of dramatic change, making it potentially less central to self. However, the framework of Piran's theory is helpful to the therapist when thinking about what needs to be different, when a younger or more mature adult has internalized some very unhelpful ideas about themselves. Here is part of an account from someone who describes her journey towards self-appreciation.

So, from being teased as a child with a spoiled face, my funny voice and haggle piggly teeth, I entered my teenage years. I was utterly convinced that no boy or man would ever love me as I was so ugly—and how I raged against the unfair-

ness of that. What resentment at feeling so cursed—it still affects me though the hold is getting less. What saved me was falling into the hands of healers and therapists (names a woman she could trust because she was also different, among others). In my thirties my self-esteem is gradually growing. I actually like scars and uneven teeth on others. But my own scar is associated with too much sorrow and resentment to fully accept it. (Female interviewee reflects on her transition to adulthood)

Difference is an additional challenge for young people to negotiate at a time when insecurities about appearance are at a peak, and older adults, reflecting on this stage describe this time as their most difficult. One older woman, now very comfortable with her appearance, kept a diary of this time (quoted above) and commented '*when I read what I had written then I was surprised at how angry and unhappy I was with how I looked. When the surgeon asked me what I wanted to have done, I just didn't know how to reply.*'

Mature Adults

Little research has been devoted to body image among older adults, although there is a reported rise in eating disorders among older women. This is in line with one of the perspectives on body ageing, which proposes that body dissatisfaction increases as ageing bodies diverge from socially accepted norms. In addition, Piran's Older Women study (2017) reports the lifelong impact of differential access. In societies focused on appearance, even compliance with norms was linked with devaluation (pretty women aren't taken seriously), and a lack of compliance incurred social penalties. Half of the sample had physical challenges, some were in poverty, they reported a lack of belief in abilities, and felt powerless to affect change.

Another seemingly contradictory perspective suggests that older adults are less concerned about body image and societal pressures lessen. Women passing menopause regularly comment on how they find themselves overlooked, suddenly invisible. Not all experience this as a bad thing—if you have been regularly evaluated as less attractive than your friends it can be a relief. One interviewee commented

I felt as if I had been excused from covert judgement on my appearance, polite avoidance and omissions and there was a greater sense of freedom. Friends I knew who had relied on their looks or felt very identified with them found ageing upsetting, disturbing to who they had thought they were. I felt a bit smug, as I had plenty of past experience to draw on (of negative stereotyping) and more confidence in other aspects of myself.

In so far as pressures are generated partially by the social group, both could be true—nobody really wants to look old (when it is defined as a lack or fading of attractiveness), but peer comparison and the skills that come with maturity ameliorate this, and many people adjust their expectations. The increase in media images of glamorous and thin older actresses and personalities may be contributing to the increase in both cosmetic surgery and eating problems among older women, as they seek to remain attractive and relevant ('still in the game'), though there is little current research so far. Another older female interviewee commented,

Post menopause I felt fine, good about myself, but as I reached 60, and in a senior role at work I felt it was quite an ageist environment. I worried that my visible difference was also more of a disadvantage then. Particularly now, there is a media-fanned culture of resenting the old. I did get some cosmetic work done, just to make myself look a bit 'fresher'. Though it didn't alter my difference, it helped me to feel more confident.

Following on from this, research on visible differences across age groups has consistently reported that the severity of problems reported by their subjects is not related to objective visible difference, with some of those with very mild problems reporting greater distress. Recent research finds that individual adjustment is related to personality variables such as optimism, as well as social support and post traumatic growth (Ong et al. 2007; Egan et al. 2011).

The psychological support offered to families and young people with visible differences has greatly increased in the last 30 years, though what is offered varies geographically, and the best practice is concentrated in specialist centres. Many GPs still lack information on what is possible, and available. The largest difference in experience is between those born before the 1980s and those born later. Many older adults report no offer of any kind of group or therapy while growing up, and most did not meet anyone who looked like them, except possibly in their ward at hospital. Those who had therapy later accessed it through their GPs. As the internet was not yet created, families were largely left to their own resources. What was available in terms of treatment was also much more limited, so adults who encounter young people with similar problems find that they have been offered many more treatment options alongside psychological support if needed and are amazed.

They reflect that this was the most painful time, but there was a culture of 'getting on with it', and little choice but to do so. So, in fact they often report beginning romantic relationships earlier, and the lack of electronic interface had some advantages. Strong communities and faith groups are named by interviewees as buffers against any stigma, though the past tendency to a 'carry on' approach to problems meant that difference was not discussed. All agree that the transition to secondary school, at a time when self-awareness was altering and sensitivity to appearance was acute, was the most difficult to negotiate. Young men who traditionally had been expected to 'make the first move' also reported that it was hard to believe that anyone would want them as a date. Typically, people waited for others to let them know, unless they had a helpful go-between. One interviewee, now a successful businessman, said that his cousin commented '*I always thought you were a bit weird, but you are alright really*', having said nothing about it throughout his childhood. Reflecting on this he mused that people did not understand his difference and were a bit afraid even if they were quite familiar. While courting his wife who had grown up as a family friend he asked for a kiss, and she turned him down. Later she told him that she was worried his scar would make kissing him strange and wondered how she would cope. Happily, she got over this, and they are still married, now with grandchildren.

If an older adult with a visible difference seeks therapy with you, the presenting issue is quite likely to be age related—bereavement, retirement, family disputes, 'legacy' or regrets, loneliness and despair, health anxiety, and so on. How do you think their personal history of difference would affect their presentation? Would you mention it if they didn't?

This difference in support offered to previous generations has now been corrected by the welcome new research initiatives, such as those now tracking all patients with visible differences through different stages. These are relatively new and will take many years to yield adult data. The 'born earlier' group is still hard to reach, with most discharged at 18 if not before. Adult research samples are mainly 'opportunity' based, relying on organisations like CLAPA and Changing Faces which have self-selecting databases.

These experienced adults are an untapped resource for the most part, but interviewees have talked about meeting people during their working or social lives who have recently welcomed a different child into the family. It is a stressful time for these new parents, with many fears about what their baby might have to face in the future. They are impressed and relieved to speak to someone who has obviously come through their difficulties and established a successful life. The message they are happy to share is 'It will be OK'.

References

Alsheikh N, Parmeswaran P, Elhoweris H (2015) Parenting style, self-esteem and student performance in the United Arab Emirates. *Current Issues in Education* 13(1):1–23

Argyle M (2008) Social encounters: contributions to social interaction. Aldine Transaction.

Baumrind D (1991) Parenting styles and adolescent development. *The Journal of Early Adolescence* 11(1):56–95

Bearman SK, Presnell K, Stice ME, (2006) The skinny on body dissatisfaction: A longitudinal study of adolescent boys and girls. *Journal of youth and adolescence* 35(2):229–241

Bourdieu (1986) The Forms of Capital. In: Richardson J (ed) Handbook of theory and research for the sociology of education. Greenwood, New York, pp 241–258

Brown S (2012) Interventions for families and health professionals. In: Rumsey N, Harcourt D (eds) The Oxford handbook of the psychology of appearance. Oxford University Press

Burnham J (2012) Developments in social GGRRRAAACCEESSS visible-invisible and voiced-unvoiced. In: Krause I-B (ed) Culture and reflexivity in systemic psychotherapy: mutual perspectives. Routledge

Butler C (2015) Intersectionality in family therapy training: inviting students to embrace the complexities of lived experience. *Journal of Family therapy* 37:583–589

Cadogan J (2010) Changing provision in healthcare settings in the United Kingdom. In: Rumsey N, Harcourt D (eds) The Oxford handbook of the psychology of appearance. Oxford University Press

Corry NH, Klick B, Fauerbach JA (2010) Post traumatic stress disorder and pain impact functioning and disability after major burn injury. *Journal of burn care and research* 31(1):13–25

Coy K, Spelz ML, Jones K (2002) Facial appearance and attachment in infants with orofacial clefts: a replication. *Cleft Palate-craniofacial Journal* 39:66–72

Crenshaw KW (1991) Mapping the Margins: Intersectionality, identity politics, and violence against women of color. Stanford Law Review 43(6):1241–1299

Dion KK (1973) Young children's stereotyping of facial attractiveness. *Developmental Psychology* 9:183–188

Egan K, Harcourt D, Rumsey N, The Appearance Research Collaboration (2011) A qualitative study of the experiences of people who identify themselves as having positively adjusted to visible difference. *Journal of Health Psychology* 16:739–749

Erikson EH (1980) Identity and the life cycle. Norton Books

Erikson EH (1985) The lifecycle completed. Norton Books

Field TM, Vega-Lahr N (1984) Early interactions between infants with craniofacial anomalies and their mothers. *Infant Behavioural Development* 7:527–530

Frederickson BL, Roberts TA, (1997) Objectification Theory: Towards understanding women's lived experiences and mental health risks. *Psychology of women quarterly* 21:173–206

Frisen A, Holmqvist K (2010) What characterizes early adolescents with a positive body image? A qualitative investigation of Swedish girls and boys. Body Image 7:205–212

Hoss RA, Langlois JH (2003) Infants prefer attractive faces. In: Pascalis O, Slater A (eds) The development of face processing in infancy and early childhood: current perspectives. Nova Science, New York, pp 27–38

Iawakuma M (2002) The body as embodiment: An investigation of the body by Merlau-Ponty In: Corker M, Shakespeare T (eds) Disability/Postmodernity.

Johanssen B , Ringsberg K (2004) Parents experiences of having a child with a cleft lip and palate. J Adv Nurs 47:165–173

Lansdown R, Rumsey N, Bradbury E, Carr T, Partridge J (1997) Visibly different: coping with disfigurement. Reed Educational and Professional Publishing Ltd

Leong V, Byrne E, Clackson K, Georgieva S, Lam S, Wass S (2017) Speaker gaze increases infant-adult connectivity PNAS; 28, published online November 2017 at www.pnas.org/cgi/Doi/10.1073/pnas

Lowes J, Tiggemann M (2003) Body dissatisfaction, dieting awareness and the impact of parental influence in young children. Br J Health Psychol 8:135–147

Marcia JE, Waterman AS, Matteson DR, Archer SL, Orlofsky JL (2012) Ego identity: a handbook for psychosocial research. Springer Science and Business Media

Maris CL, Endriga MC, Jones K, De Klyen M (2000) Are infants with orofacial clefts at risk for insecure mother-child attachments? *Cleft Palate-Craniofacial Journal* 37:257–265

Nash JC (2008) Rethinking intersectionality. *Feminist Review* 89:1–15

Ong J, Clarke A, White P, Johnson M, Withey S, Butler PEM (2007) Does severity predict distress? The relationship between subjective and objective measures of distress and psychological adjustment, during treatment for facial lipoatrophy. Body Image 4(3):239–248

Partridge J (1990) Changing faces, a changing faces publication. ChangingFaces.org

Piran N (2017) Journeys of embodiment at the intersection of body and culture: the developmental theory of embodiment, 1st edn. Elsevier

Ramsay JL, Langlois JH, (2002) Effects of the 'beauty is good' stereotype on children's information processing. *Journal of Experimental Child Psychology* 81:320–340

Robinson E (1997) Psychological research on visible difference in adults. In: Lansdown R, Rumsey N, Bradbury E, Carr T, Partridge J (eds) Visibly different: coping with disfigurement. Butterworth-Heinemann, Oxford, pp 102–111

Slater A, Quinn P, Hayes C, Brown E (2000) Newborn infants' preference for attractive faces: the role of internal and external facial features. Infancy 1:265–274

Smolak L (2010) Body image development in children. In: Cash TF, Smolak L (eds) Body image: a handbook of science, practice, and prevention, 2nd edn. Guildford, New York

Smolak L (2012) Appearance in childhood and adolescence. In: Rumsey N, Harcourt D (eds) The Oxford handbook of the psychology of appearance. Oxford University Press

Weilage M, Hope DA, (1999) Self-discrepancy in social phobia and dysthymia. *Cognitive therapy and research* 23:637–650

4

The Family Context

The dance between self and others through which we understand our-selves can sometimes feel complicated, occasionally more like a battle, but across the world the family context is important. In countries with a diverse population in the twenty-first century the meaning of the word 'family' needs to be expanded to include multi-generation households, stepfamilies, later life families, same-sex couples with children, families with mixed ethnicity and cultures and families of ethnic minorities, who may have important members living elsewhere. It is hard, or maybe impossible, for one word to contain all it needs to in this situation, but the wish for a 'good' family, and respect, pride (or shame) in our origins, though it may not define us as adults, continues. The resilience of the 'family' grouping as an efficient 'change and continuity machine' is being tested as never before by migration and globalisation. In each family con-figuration the critical issues of power, belief, meaning (and who or what defines it), gender, intimacy, integrity, resilience and capacity for change need to be held in mind when thinking about the individual in relation to the group. A professional commitment to social justice, ethical stan-dards and human rights can guide therapists in this complex environ-ment (see Harvard's Pluralism project http://pluralism.org).

© The Author(s) 2020
V. Purcell, *Understanding Visible Differences*, Palgrave Texts in Counselling and
Psychotherapy, https://doi.org/10.1007/978-3-030-51655-0_4

> When assessing a new client how much attention do you give to mapping their family network? What does your choice mean about your practice?

While earlier life cycle models assumed a sequential progression, then more likely to be the social norm, contemporary life-span research recognises the possibility of diverse and fluid relational patterns over the life course (Walsh 2012). Though the course is more varied, the majority still hope to establish a committed relationship, and most still wish to be parents, though the first is not necessarily a given for the second. For the therapist a position of curiosity and not-knowing in their attempt to understand the experience of their clients is really the only viable option. Drawing a 'map' or chart of important others is a useful way to begin to unpick meanings which may be unhelpfully submerged or entrenched. Many of our clients, presenting with anxiety, depression, trauma or interpersonal problems have lost interest in themselves, or become frustrated at their perceived failures. The therapist's interest and respect is an invitation to alter their perspective and regard unspoken thoughts and feelings with interest.

> Family beliefs are absorbed, forming the fabric of verbal and non-verbal communications, and as such are powerful but not always immediately available for scrutiny. How easy or difficult is it for your client to make choices based on their own beliefs rather than family rules?

Visible Difference and Family Life

A visibly different child arrives into a home with even greater impact than a 'normal' child, because of the attendant medical needs. The opportunity to recognise and effectively process this impact on mothers and family members varies greatly, depending on the resources available, and research has not yet offered clear answers as to the exact role of the family in the development and maintenance of body dis/satisfaction. However, Bellew (2012) reports that a likely model is emerging in which the family offers information in the first instance, and interpretation of social and cultural messages. Ideally this transmission of information and understanding takes place in a stable and beneficial environment. In real life there is often the need to backtrack, check, embrace, correct, protect, sometimes apologise and forgive when things have gone awry.

> Ways of resolving problems in relation to conflict or difficulty are also learned in the family context. How might this be helping or hindering your client?

The very limited research available to date suggests that the family milieu contributes more strongly to appearance adjustment in childhood, and values related to appearance are later modified in adolescence and adulthood within friendship and romantic relationships.

In the case of a newborn with visible difference, where there are other children in the family an explanation needs to be offered which is non-stigmatising, age appropriate and facilitative of adjustments that need to be made for medical interventions. Families with a strong faith can draw much from their spirituality to find strength and resilience, but any explanation for difference which implies that punishment from god or spirit energy has been enacted on the child (or parent) is particularly unhelpful. Where these views are likely to be held by their faith group or members of the wider family, this needs to be carefully re-interpreted and managed to protect the children's self-esteem. Walsh (2010) comments that '*in family life, patriarchal precepts have been used to justify the denigration and abuse of wives and children … therapists have an ethical responsibility to address denigrating and abusive behaviour, whether rooted in family, ethnic, or religious beliefs and traditions*'.

> Do you have clinical experiences of this kind of context? How did you deal with it? Do you have colleagues that you can discuss these issues with, without judgement or repercussions?

Sibling Issues

The age and stages of the other children matter, and the risk of them being or feeling sidelined by the urgent medical needs of the new sibling are immediate. Resentment about the loss of attention and normal family life, and fears and fantasies of what might have caused the trauma, for instance a mistaken idea that they may have contributed to it in some way, are some of the difficulties identified by Barlow and Ellard (2006). This is very well illustrated in the recent film 'Wonder' (2017) in which Via, the older sister, struggles in transition to a new school despite her love for her brother, and for a time pretends that she is an only child to avoid complications.

Again, the research on family impact has mixed results, with some meta-analytic studies finding that siblings are at greater risk of anxiety and/or depression because of internalised feelings, or alternatively of expressing them through oppositional or aggressive behaviours. The analysis also found greater instances of low self-esteem, and individual, family and school related problems among siblings (Vermaes et al. 2012). This is an additional challenge for families already stretched by a new arrival. But taking the time to talk and listen to the children and include them as much as possible will mean that problems do not develop 'under the radar'.

> It is particularly difficult for parents to acknowledge the problems of older children when they are struggling to adjust to a different child. Good wider family networks can be helpful here, and if your client remembers strong support from a grandparent or other relative it may be worth wondering with them about what was happening at that time.

In a study involving children with cancer the researchers reported that positive sibling adjustment was associated with resilience, self-esteem, empathy, pro-social behaviours, assertiveness, increased family cohesion and an expressive family environment (Alderfer et al. 2014; Barlow and Ellard 2006). This emphasises the importance of ensuring that the other children adjust well to the new arrival so that the sibling network develops in resilience. Concern for the risk to these children's wellbeing has led to the development of specific family-oriented groups for well siblings by some charities, and research finds that these and broad spectrum psychosocial programmes are associated with better family outcomes.

Solving Things Together

The adjustments families need to make depend greatly on the nature of the difficulty and will vary over the course of development. Characteristically, healthy family systems have good problem-solving skills and use them successfully around each challenge, enabling growth and change. The important message for all the children here is that things can be difficult at times, but by working together and dealing with issues, problems can be managed. So, explaining and including them in an age-appropriate way helps them build their own sense of competence. When there is a crisis elsewhere in the family, for instance divorce or parental illness extra support may be needed. For a therapist, a genogram or 'map' of who is considered as the family (whether a relative or friend) and other related support systems is very helpful. This may include a specialist health team if longer term intervention has been needed, or other support groups. For siblings, as well as those who are different, there is also the opportunity for psychological enrichment and the development of resilience and compassion through the challenges they experience.

Facing Up to Bullying

Children are more likely to be bullied when they are vulnerable in some way, and support organisations report that children who are visibly different and/or disabled are two to three times as likely to be subjected to this at some time. For parents of a newborn child with visible difference this is often one of their worst fears and can create strong feelings of guilt when thinking about struggles their child might face in the future. There is consistent research to show that bullying within the family or at school has negative consequences for the victim which can continue long into adult life. It often begins when the child does not have the cognitive architecture to understand what is happening and why. Therefore, it is important that both siblings and index child are aware of what bullying and scapegoating is (where one person attempts to degrade, abuse or control a less powerful person) what to do, and the importance of telling.

> As a parent how would you talk about this, with children of different ages?

With helpful intervention a sibling network can be a wonderful system for learning how to manage power and recognise its occasional misuse. Taking a systemic non-judgmental perspective can help all of them express what they feel and manage what they do in a better way. It is intensely painful for parents to know that their child is having these experiences, and they may need to intervene if (for instance) the school fails to. The support of others who have encountered similar situations is invaluable, and although these are undeniably difficult to handle, with non-judgmental help children can develop wisdom and sensitivity to other's feelings beyond their years.

> Being able to suggest a few different resources to try can be very useful, some will appeal more, and be more helpful than others.

In the internet age there are many resources available, such as personal accounts of being bullied and how to deal with it online. See #LifeIsACatwalk for video of young people 'walking' in the 2018 Autumn Collection show of designer Steven Tai. This event was also featured by Glamour, Vogue India and the BBC News. One of the models also appeared on channel 5 news talking about her experience of being bullied after she suddenly lost all her hair at a very young age. She describes how she and her wig were the target of abuse at school, on one occasion it was even taken and flushed down the loo. Now she is a confident, beautiful and articulate young woman, who appears comfortable with her identity and baldness. The photographer Rankin made portraits of the participants, which will be published in collaboration with the charity Changing Faces @FaceEquality. Their inspiring accounts, and confidence that they do not need to hide and can achieve much is an inspiration to children struggling with prejudice in the playground.

If children of the same family later attend the same school, there may be a responsibility on some to protect others which also needs to be considered and monitored carefully. There are several online resources now available for parents concerned about this, and one of the largest can be accessed via Bullying UK, and Family Lives (previously Parentline). They offer online parenting courses, a confidential helpline and the chance to chat online with other parents.

Doing It Well Enough

Beavers and Hampson (2003) found in their study of family functioning that no single factor differentiated well-functioning from dysfunctional families. Instead, they drew attention to many aspects of strength and vulnerability, taking a multi-system perspective. From extensive clinical work and research Walsh (2016) identifies key processes in family resilience, and they are grouped into three main areas—family belief systems, communication processes and organisational processes. No child or family exists in isolation, so beyond the child/family group, community and sociocultural belief systems, communication processes, and organisational processes also impact, and for the developing older child and adolescent these become increasingly important. For a further discussion of these issues, see Walsh (2016).

> While each family has a particular style, a pattern which includes regular ways of talking and listening is helpful. Where the family style is not talking about things, how much does your client wish to change this? What might help?

Walsh helpfully reminds us that 'normal' families are not problem free, any more than 'normal' lives are. Confidence comes from the ability to manage adversity and change in ways that strengthen the positive and increase resilience. Also, from being able to admit when it is hard, and give appropriate expression to feelings. Sometimes it is not necessary (or possible) to change others, but as a member of the system thinking and behaving differently has the potential to change the 'possibility field' of the group. Being able to speak about difference to each other within the family is a place for this to begin. Acknowledging the existence of prejudice in some social situations is likely to create a space in which even the most difficult experiences can be spoken about. The advent of #metoo in 2017 has made everyone more aware that often those who suffer abuse also feel shame and are reluctant to talk about it. Children and young people need help from family, friends and school to manage the challenges of socialising successfully, as discussed in the previous chapter. The early establishment of a sense of self-worth not based primarily on appearance gives a robust basis to face the complexities of interaction with the wider social world.

Peer-Related Issues

Until recently the research on visible differences in children and young people has focused mainly on the role of peer relationships, largely driven by a negative, pathologising view. Much appearance research has also taken a broader perspective with a focus on body image and eating behaviour (Rumsey and Harcourt 2017). What specific research has been published tends to focus on one disfigurement type and burn patient samples are currently over-represented. Robinson (1997) reports that studies of other forms of disfigurement tend to have smaller samples drawn from hospital-based research. Though this is improving there is little funding, so samples tend to be opportunity-based, limiting the conclusions which can be drawn. There is a general agreement that the social isolation and stigma experienced is objectively real and related to prejudice towards those with unusual appearances. Problems with social anxiety, negative self-image, depression and avoidance increase in adolescence as young people become more self-conscious. Harter (2003) found that by middle school body esteem was a component of general self-esteem. The direction of this relationship is still debated with contradicting research findings. The relationship between body esteem and depression is clearer, with Stice and Bearman (2001) finding that negative body image at least partly predicts depressive symptoms in girls and suggesting that the difference between boys' and girls' body dissatisfaction accounted for the higher incidence of depression in girls.

How would you approach trying to help a depressed young girl with a visible difference referred for therapy?

There is an abundance of anecdotal and research evidence which shows that many young people spend an increased amount of time on appearance—related conversation, including 'fat talk' (Jones et al. 2018). Jones found that these interactions are associated with poorer body image for both sexes. Among girls these conversations can be complicated for those with a visible difference, who wonder at the minutia of these anxieties, and what their friends really think of them. The friends can also find it complicated, sometimes commenting that they are 'oversensitive'. The influence of family wanes at this time, but older siblings are more likely to be included in the conversation if the age gap is not too wide and can help to give perspective. The importance of peers who can share similar experiences also increases, and online groups, summer camps and media stories are more accessible.

These can lead to helpful discussion of how to cope with social bullying, feelings of failure and exclusion. Anger, possible misinterpretation and blame-giving can also be acknowledged and age-appropriate discussions about difference given. However, it is important to note again that the severity of the physical difference is not a predictor of difficulty, and some report that their disfigurement plays a minor role in their lives. For example, Blakeney et al. (1988) assessed a sample of young people with facial burn injuries, finding that they were well adjusted psychologically compared with others of a similar age. Important factors are the support of family and friend networks, and explicit and implicit messages available to make sense of their experience.

Parents Who Struggle

Nobody gets to choose their family. This works both ways, and most therapists can recall clients who say they felt 'like cuckoos in the nest'. Parents don't choose which child they get either, and a few very honest ones may say they don't like their children. Whatever complexities this summarises, it can be a problem.

Most parents want to do their best for their children, but of course whether their child is able-bodied or not there is a small proportion who struggle to form a stable attachment, reject their child or give very inconsistent care. This environment contributes to poor outcomes for the child in the short and medium term without early intervention from health and mental health professionals. Parental rejection and criticism increases the risk of behavioural and interpersonal problems (Rohner et al. 2008). Perceived parental rejection is also associated with attachment problems in intimate relationships in adulthood. It is not a well-researched area in relation to visible differences, but signs of attachment problems will be similar in all children (and adults).

> What can you do if the family unit is resistant to intervention by professionals? How would you attempt to create a window of hope for your client? Sometimes this can be done by story, or example.

Even when the family is basically loving and supportive problems can arise which make coping difficult. Where differences are congenital, some more stable families rarely talk about difference, if ever, if this type of communication is not part of the family culture. If there are mental health problems with one parent, difficulties increase. One middle aged interviewee recalled

I had a "nervous breakdown" at 9, it was the situation at home. My father had anxiety problems and he would just erupt, looking back it didn't feel like a safe haven. Food was an issue, and I didn't eat for about 6 weeks. My mum took me to the doctor but told me not to talk about what was going on at home, in case they broke up the family. I felt I was weak and less able to cope, and people said "she's highly strung". My difference was never discussed, it was always "please don't make a fuss". My sisters are still like that if I mention anything. … It was years later I realised that choking when I was very small, because of congenital feeding difficulties had an impact. I never ate meat. It took much longer to understand my strengths.

After working through her problems with a counsellor when she was in her 30s she later became someone able to help others.

What Therapists Can Contribute to Family Systems and Support: Some Examples

Kindsvatter et al. (2013) recommend the use of therapeutic letters in working with parents and children to improve relationships. Responses to attachment insecurity include hyperactivation—with the seeking of proximity, attention and reassurance, or alternatively deactivation— where the child achieves and seeks to maintain distance, has a dismissive or angry stance and can be defensive in anticipation of rejection. The team use brief letters, 4–5 paragraphs long, which are sent to clients between sessions giving permanency and consistency to messages thera- pists wish to emphasise. Firstly, there are letters of engagement with the dismissive parent, followed by letters of explanation which acknowledge the parent's own experiences of being unheard or neglected. Following this, as treatment progresses there are letters of change which acknowl- edge and affirm progress. A fuller description of the approach can be found in the referenced paper.

> If letters are not part of your clinic's treatment model a well written assess- ment and/or discharge letter can still be powerful. It is surprising how often these are kept for years by clients, especially those who have not previously felt seen or heard.

If, after a relatively normal early life trauma leaves one or more family members with an enduring visible difference and/or disability this is a rupture in the previous family story, one which may require additional resources and possibly attitude change from other members. The abrupt- ness of change is a factor in itself. Rolland (2018), writing about the experience of illness and disability in the family comments 'Social stigma is an important cause of disability in many disorders. For instance, cere- bral palsy, severe burns, or psoriasis are cosmetically disabling and dis- torting of body image to the extent that the attendant social stigma interferes with normal social interaction. Often treatment procedures produce psychosocial difficulties because of disfiguration.' This shocking alteration in status can result in a period where the person (or family) appears to be frozen, or suspended in time, and unable to engage with the tasks needed to adapt to their new circumstances, an indicator that extra support is needed.

A Brief Case Example: Losing 'Value' and Getting It Back

A young woman with a 'traditional' Middle Eastern migrant background sought treatment for depression on the advice of her doctor after an accident at work. The resulting small scar on her face had caused her to feel unable to return to work, and she felt ashamed that she had been stupid enough to cause the accident. She did not want to be seen, rarely left her flat, avoided previously enjoyed activities, and former friends. In fact, it was as if her outside life had just stopped. She explained that in her culture a woman's facial features were very important, and she felt that her scar meant she had no future, as no-one would want to marry her. The therapist struggled to engage her in the recommended treatment, and brought her case to supervision. We agreed that the therapist needed to support her in a period of mourning the person she saw herself as, and the future she believed she would have, before beginning the process of helping her go out into the world and live her life as she was now.

Although her family was traditional in their plans for her, in some respects she was a modern city woman, trying to achieve a successful balance between different value systems. The therapist spent time helping her recognise the ways that she had already helped the family to adapt by choosing her studies, working, and in her friendships. The next step was to explore her fears about what might happen if someone noticed her scar, and role play how to manage this. It was agreed that she could draw attention to it in the conversation, as waiting and wondering if they had noticed would be stressful. Eventually she felt ready to take the risk, and despite her negative predictions was very surprised by how easy it was, encouraging her to continue to experiment. The reactions she had expected did not happen, and before ending treatment she reported that she felt she was a stronger person after coming through her trauma.

This was a great outcome, and while it is always possible to improve coping skills it would be unrealistic to expect that circumstances always permit immediate improvement, or to set unreasonable goals which reinforce feelings of failure. Her story underlines the research finding that severity does not predict adjustment ability. Families may have multiple problems, including poverty of communication and resources, which challenge the client and therapist. In some circumstances improvement may be slow with relapses due to limited material and emotional capacity. Support may be best found outside the family system, particularly in a therapy space which allows the opportunity for safe experimentation. As always, part of the treatment is to help the client think about how to cope with future difficulties before ending.

One dramatic difference between congenital and acquired difference is that the first may be 'normalised' and largely subsumed in familiar contexts, whereas the dramatic change of acquired difference is more likely to be talked about, and resources gathered to cope with change. A family group which is flexible and resourced enough can shift focus as needed, acting as a 'holding' environment, though this will not be without costs. For the index person this may mean they feel distress or guilt on seeing what other family members go through. A supportive network creates the opportunity to co-construct an adapted 'success story'—a resilient life script which refuses or moves beyond the victim narrative.

Building Resilience

Lia and Abela (2016) report on the family process of resilient individuals with acquired disability. They found that families played a vital role in the rehabilitation process, with 'virtuous circles of empathy and support'. Where that is challenged, they found that the therapist can play a crucial role in amplifying virtuous and feedback processes using narrative strategies, reframing and the creation of helpful dialogic experiences. They recommend that an expanded view of family impact and family resources should be considered when subject to health threats. Approaches should be strength focused to instil a sense of hope and belief in their potential and ability to thrive.

Again, it is not always straightforward, and Rossi et al. (2005) explore relatives' shameful feelings of guilt, blame and shame, concerning burns patients. They found an often overlooked problem that can lead to psychological issues, stress, PTSD and depression for the patient without support from health professionals. Shame can be shared and communicated, as relatives find it difficult to be with the burned person in public, who then see themselves as flawed and vulnerable. Kornhaber et al. (2018) explored the impact of these emotions cross-culturally in a systematic review and found that in some cultures the apportioning of blame and loss of face was an issue, while for others problems with creating a new identity and social rejection were more important.

In these contexts a powerful story, which does not imply blame to the individuals struggling, can serve to break through. Where the narrative found originates in that culture, perhaps in a different context, even more so.

Systemic therapists reflecting on the impact of illness on the family emphasise the importance of considering the life stage tasks and expectations of each family member when thinking about the resources available to cope with additional challenges. Levinson's work on the life course (1986) explores the way that periods of stability, continuity and stasis are interwoven with periods of change, discontinuity and fluctuation. He also argued that all aspects of living need to be considered, including inner wishes and fantasies, love relationships, involvement in family, work and other social systems, body changes, and periods when things go well or badly. Levinson uses the metaphor of the seasons when considering life stages, but other theorists argue that the family group history in relation to disfigurement or illness is an important point of reference as well. Psychological tasks may not have been completed at the time, and there may be a need among some or all members of the group to repeat or reverse an illness narrative from that history.

Once again, the use of books, soap opera characters or films as reference or discussion points can be very useful.

The view of the family as a system moving through time, with centripetal and centrifugal stages in family development (Carter and McGoldrick 1988), is helpful when considering the different challenges that all members may face and identifying where expected progression has been interrupted by trauma or stable difference. A centripetal stage is one where the natural focus is within the family, for instance during childbirth and raising younger children. In contrast, an example of a centrifugal stage would be adolescence and the transition to university and young adulthood beyond close family boundaries.

Case Example: Making the Transition to Independence with Disability

The challenges for a parent in supporting a different child to fulfil their potential are significant, especially when resources in the community are limited. In Mary's case her mother had worked tremendously hard to establish opportunities for her daughter and encourage her to do everything she possibly could, even though Mary was only mobile on crutches. To her credit the Mary I met was a highly motivated, ambitious, intelligent and active young woman, who insisted on taking the stairs despite her difficulties, never the lift. She arrived in my office to talk about her relationship with her mother, around which she had some very difficult feelings she needed to air in safety. She felt angry, entangled, unable to move on into young adulthood as her siblings had done and felt that her mother was not willing to let her go. She was the last child to leave the nest, and her mother had built a significant part of her own identity around supporting her and campaigning for resources. We met at different times over the years of her studies to talk about how she was managing the delicate transition for both her and her mother to the new stage in their relationship. It was not without storms, abortive experiments and real risk to the relationship, but over time and eventually together they negotiated their way through all the changes needed to allow Mary the space to take risks in the next stage of her life.

Some types of visible difference are analogous in certain respects to a constant course illness, where an initial event occurs, possibly involving both drama and adjustment for all members of the family group, after which the biological course stabilises. If the illness is disabling, the later stages of development may be partially altered, as in the case where the young person needs continued support and cannot live independently. This may lead to feelings of guilt on all sides, fears of being a burden for the disabled child, and a loss of expected freedoms for the parents. If the family also has an able-bodied child they may struggle to achieve full independence, due to additional caring responsibilities or guilt at having life chances their sibling cannot. Alternatively, a family that becomes enmeshed and too organised around the disability could be reluctant to let their disabled adult child to take risks, explore their limitations, and challenge themselves or live independently. The able-bodied adult child may continue to feel overlooked, and in the worst-case scenario may create a crisis as a vehicle to express this.

Even when the parent/child relationship is loving and supportive the disabled young person (or sibling) can benefit from a 'safe space' like university counselling to work out their identity and future goals. This includes a consideration of how to talk about changes with their parents, who will not be witnessing their new experiences. In each case the therapeutic task is to understand what might be 'stuck' and where the opportunities for growth and change are. It is beyond the scope of this chapter to list all possible elements in a complex network, which need to be mapped and considered carefully. Further research/enquiries/conversations may also be needed between your client and other members of the group over time to understand and help the system adjust.

References

Alderfer M, Stanley C, Conroy R, Long K, Fairclough D, Kazak A, et al (2014) The social functioning of siblings of children with cancers: a multi-informant investigation. *Journal of Paediatric Psychology* 40(3):309–319

Barlow JH, Ellard DR (2006) The psychosocial well-being of children with chronic disease, their parents and siblings: an overview of the research evidence base. *Child, Care, Health and Development* 32:19–31

Beavers WR, Hampson RB (2003) Measuring family competence: the beavers system model. In: Walsh F (ed) Normal family processes, 3rd edn. Guildford Press, New York, pp 549–580.

Bellew R (2012) The role of the family. In: The Oxford handbook of the psychology of appearance. Oxford University Press

Blakeney P, Herndon D, Desai M et al (1988) Long term psychosocial adjustment following burn injury. *Journal of Burn Care Rehabilitation* 9:661–665

Carter B, McGoldrick M (eds) (1988) The changing family lifecycle, 2nd edn. Gardner Press, New York.

Harter S (2003) The development of self-representations in childhood and adolescence. In: Leary MR, Tangney JP (eds) Handbook of self and identity. Guildford, New York, pp 610–642.

Jones M, Crowther H, Ciesla J (2018) A naturalistic study of fat talk and its behavioural and affective consequences. Body Image 11(4):337–345.

Kindsvatter A, Desmond K, Yanikoski A, Stahl S (2013) The use of therapeutic letters in addressing parent-child attachment problems. *The Family Journal: Counselling and therapy for couples and families* 21(1):74–79

Kornhaber R, Childs C, Cleary M (2018) Experiences of guilt, shame and blame in those affected by burns: a systematic review. Burns 44:1026–1039.

Levinson DJ (1986) A conception of adult development. Am Psychol 41:3–13

Lia ES, Abela A, (2016) Not broken, but strengthened: stories of resilience by persons with acquired physical disability and their families. *Australia and New Zealand Journal of Family Therapy* 37:400–417

Robinson E (1997) Psychological research on visible difference in adults. In: Lansdown R, Rumsey N, Bradbury E, Carr T, Partridge J (eds) Visibly different: coping with disfigurement. Butterworth-Heinemann, Oxford, pp 102–111.

Rohner RP, Khaleque A, Cournoyer D (2008) Parental acceptance-rejection: theory, methods, cross-cultural evidence and implications. Ethos 3(3):299–334.

Rolland JS (2018) Helping couples and families navigate illness and disability: an integrated approach. Guildford Press, London, New York.

Rossi LA, Villa Vda S, Zago MM, Ferreira E (2005) The stigma of burns perception of burned patient's relatives when facing discharge from hospital. Burns 31:37–44.

Rumsey N, Harcourt D (eds) (2017) The Oxford handbook of the psychology of appearance. Oxford University Press, Oxford.

Stice E, Bearman SK (2001) Body image and eating disturbances prospectively predict increases in depressive symptoms in adolescent girls: a growth curve analysis. Dev Psychol 37:597–607

Vermaes IP, van Susante AM, and van Bakel HJ (2012) Psychological functioning of siblings in children with chronic health conditions. *Journal of Paediatric Psychology* 37(1):66–184

Walsh F. (2010) Spiritual Diversity: Multifaith perspectives in family therapy. *Family Process* 49(3):30–348

Walsh F (2012) The 'New Normal': diversity and complexity in twenty first century families. In: Walsh F (ed) Normal family processes, 4th edn. Guildford Press, New York, pp 4–27.

Walsh F (2016) Strengthening family resilience, 3rd edn. Guildford Press, New York.

5

Relationships: Outside of the Family Group

This chapter is divided into two sections, to provide structure for the wide range of experiences covered.

Part 1: Dealing with Difference in Friendship, Love and Work

'Be what you are and say what you feel because those who mind don't matter, and those who matter don't mind.' *Dr Seuss*

This new set of challenges begins when the child goes to their first school, and encounters others from different backgrounds, mainly without the mediating presence of family. All children at this stage will have a restricted range of social skills, but as noted in the previous chapter, they also already have preferences for certain faces. The surrounding adults can really help by being aware of this already formed bias and preparing the different child for the experience of curious questioning and dealing with comments. If the family has a way of talking about the experiences of hospital visits, scars and other things this can be done without causing anxiety about 'new people'.

© The Author(s) 2020
V. Purcell, *Understanding Visible Differences*, Palgrave Texts in Counselling and
Psychotherapy, https://doi.org/10.1007/978-3-030-51655-0_5

> Talking about a child's differences, their possible impact on others, and the meanings of that, as well as how to manage them is very important. Especially when the differences are facial. It is very hard for parents sometimes, connecting as it does with their own anxieties. At best it should be routine, appropriate and normal.

There are many parent discussions online, and resources are available to help (Department of Education 2014). The school can be advised in advance, so that they have considered how to manage a successful integration and if needed offer age-appropriate corrective interventions if a child is picked on. It is helpful if the new children they encounter have skilled helpers with diversity training, but this is not always the case. Parents are advised to meet their new school teacher beforehand if possible. If not, an example of an introductory letter for parents to send prior to their child starting school is given by the American Children's Craniofacial Organisation (for instance) and is available online.

Active Strategies to Reduce Stigma and Create Supporters

Reading and talking about stories at circle time is a simple way of introducing new ideas and encouraging children to develop their understanding and acceptance of difference, which can cover a range of things from size, appearance, skin colour and accent. In some infant and primary schools parents are encouraged to help with activities, and this offers them a chance to make a difference (with the teacher's agreement). Though there is currently little good research to indicate which of the many possible approaches is best, the need to provide materials and help teachers feel comfortable introducing children to diversity and good values in a multicultural society is very apparent. An internet search for 'children's storybooks about being different' will yield many results, and some are great classics, like 'Elmer' the elephant, 'Dr. Seuss' 'The Sneetches'. More recent ones include 'Giraffes can't Dance', 'Break the Mould' and 'The Five of Us' by Quentin Blake, all of which could lead easily to a discussion about accepting and valuing those who are different.

Interestingly, if you substitute 'diversity' for difference in the same search there is little overlap in the titles found, with a much greater focus on single ethnic groups rather than a general valuing of difference. A range of resources can only be helpful and there is a growing need to focus on inclusivity, for the benefit of communities.

> Many UK primary schools welcome parent support with reading, and if the family is supported by a charity they may welcome this involvement too.

To support nurseries and parents the UK government has issued guidelines on equality and diversity in early years learning, and visible difference is now considered a 'protected characteristic.' Practice guidelines for those working in the field cover gender, age, sexual orientation, race and ethnicity, language and culture, faith and belief, and ability. (O'Connor 2018) Visible difference, including weight, should be understood as something that can cause difficulties not because of the difference but the ways people see them, and institutions provide for them. There is some evidence though that the intelligence of children who are visibly different is often underestimated, and they can suffer from the 'soft prejudice' of low expectations, leading to under-performance. On entering school parents may need to make it clear that their child has no cognitive impairment if this might be the case.

Naming Problem Behaviours and Focusing on Anti-Bullying

Differences in appearance have been linked with peer relationship difficulties and bullying (Vannatta et al. 2009). Children and young people need the opportunity to talk about these experiences as an individual, work out their own strategies to deal with them and have the support of adults. Bradbury (1997) comments that *'individuals can be helped to become "experts" in handling social situations, by treating the problems as familiar and understandable, and by exploring and developing ways of interacting with others'*. Alongside this a whole school approach to tolerating difference and valuing diversity has been found to be effective for both children with visible differences and other children, though it needs to be implemented by all staff.

> Reduced interest and engagement with school can be an indicator of subtle bullying, similarly a decline in achievement. Having a skill, interest or talent in a particular area which can be encouraged is a great antidote.

Anecdotal accounts from adults regularly identify early school years as a time when bullying first happened and self-confidence was undermined. On the other hand, words and actions at this time can be significant and memorable. One interviewee recalls '*there wasn't much what I would call full-out bullying, you know, pinned in a corner ... but there were a few incidents early on*'. She goes on to say that her father helped her by explaining how 'people evolved from animals, and they still have those basic instincts, to hold back from those not like them, for safety. Sometimes it helps to remove the ignorance, ask a question- like 'would you like to know what happened?' She found out later that there was a whole school assembly without her, to explain and improve children's behaviour. After that the girls who had at first been her persecutors took her under their wing and became friends.

> Peers need to know that a child's difference is not the most important, relevant or interesting thing about them.

Siblings can also be a great source of support if needed, and are sometimes easier to confide in. They often feel strongly protective as media personality Carol Vorderman comments, recalling the stares her brother Anton got while they were children '*I used to feel very angry when people stared rudely at him when we were out. ... Anton didn't talk about his feelings back then-you didn't. It was more about shutting up and getting on with it. But growing up with him did change my attitude to appearance. Today we are so obsessed with looks and I don't get that*' (Daily Mail, 14 June 2009). He later went on to become a successful businessman and advocate for others.

Support from Others with Similar Experiences

This can be a worrying time for parents, and support groups can make a real difference in providing ideas and inspiration. One parent, commenting online about how 'Augie' in R.J. Palacio's novel 'Wonder' (Palacio 2012) had helped his young son, picked out the character's comment that *'If I found a magic lamp and I could have one wish, I would wish that I had a normal face that no-one noticed at all'*. He then says that his son wishes for the exact same thing every time he is asked that question and adds 'while I would like that mainstream acceptance for Peter, I also believe he has a unique opportunity to leave others with a life-altering impression (ccakids.org). The novel and film had a big impact, though some commentators have found the sentiments difficult, calling it *'inspiration porn'* and *'feelgood for normals'*.

This loving father's comment may be true, but it is a big task for a small child whose longing to just fit in and be like everyone else is profound, especially in earlier years. It is not surprising that there are difficult times as well as occasions when they are relaxed and happy. Different children may rarely meet others like themselves, and these opportunities are important to help them understand, accept and value who they are. Summer camps are fun, and support groups can also offer chances for parents and children to meet for things like picnics. With the rise of social media, it is easier to maintain these connections, and continue to share experiences as social life becomes more complicated. One young interviewee comments *'my best friend and I met at a charity picnic and she has the same difference as me, we have been friends since then and I can talk to her about anything.'* Working out your relationship with the 'normal' others, and your sexual identity, or just having the courage to show a romantic interest in someone else can feel very risky for any young person, and these issues often start in primary school.

What opportunities has your client previously had in this respect?

Many older children would also respond differently to the wish expressed by Augie, and might feel offended by the assumption that they just want to look normal. At this later stage it could feel like a devaluing of an important part of themselves they have worked to embrace. This may have been created in part by having to deal with some very difficult experiences, including surgery, at a time when other children are still wanting to 'fit in', giving them a different perspective. Sometimes though it can feel necessary to 'park' these emotional challenges. As another interviewee commented '*I couldn't cope with comments about my appearance then, or talk about it, I was very sensitive.*' At this time she felt that avoidance and deflection were her friends, but looking back realises that having a trusted peer group would have made a big difference.

> Friendships at this stage are often about shared likes, humour and interests, and these can be fostered by caring adults.

Sudden Changes in Appearance

Children who suddenly become visibly different can find that their previously reliable ways of interacting socially don't work well any more, and they are confronted by a steep social learning curve on re-integration post-treatment. One commented '*I came across as overconfident and brash. It's overcompensation. If you are pretty you forget how much you use that as a form of communication. … Now I have to rely on my personality*' (Wheatley 1993, in Lansdown et al. 1997). It takes time for people to get to know your personality though, and a more nuanced understanding of how others react to you is needed, in addition to the toughness to manage rude and intrusive behaviour at times. The thoughtless or curious responses of strangers can mean the everyday privacy others take for granted is not afforded. This high visibility can lead to feelings of vulnerability and emotional harm, in turn causing social avoidance. Learning to cope requires a higher level of social awareness and skill, and paradoxically this can mean they have less shared experience in common with their 'visibly normal' peers. In most cases prejudice consists of a network of out-of-awareness, unchallenged assumptions, which just seem to be 'the way things are'.

Shared interests and contributing to success in teams can be a way to over-come this, provided that the opportunities are created.

More Sources of Help, Inspiration and Information

The UK charity Changing Faces provides a schools service offering phone and face-to-face contact with the young person and school staff, plus a range of education packs, PowerPoint presentations, lesson plans, activity sheets and other resources which aim to promote inclusive classroom environments. There have been assessments of the effectiveness of differ-ent versions of these interventions (Cline et al. 1998; Stock and Whale 2011). While these did not show conclusive improvements in attitude, this appears to be because pre-intervention measures indicated high levels of awareness and acceptance. The intervention was well received and atti-tudes towards visible difference very positive.

In addition to materials for use in schools Changing Faces (2010) offers online resources and phone support to help children and young people with strategies to manage conversations about difference with their peers and others.

Children with facial differences may have several surgical interventions as their face grows and changes. This often requires a period away from school, and unusual shifts in appearance which need to be managed on their return.

As understanding of the socially constructed challenges faced by peo-ple with visible differences has grown efforts have been made to ensure that a psychologist is attached to surgical teams to provide support. This includes social skills training for patients undergoing corrective surgeries. Evaluation of this provision (Kish and Lansdown 2000) indicates that the model is helpful, enhancing coping skills and improving confidence. Skills need to be acquired for different social contexts though, and an interview- based study with people disfigured by cancer of the face and neck found variation in comfort levels between small and large groups with some participants always comfortable whatever the size of group, and others occasionally so depending on the context (Bonnano and Choi 2010). Children and young people who have developed confidence in one school setting may struggle after the transition to secondary school or university.

Case Example: Changing Schools

A very clear example of this is given in this (anonymised) summary of mov-ing from middle to senior school by a girl who says *'in middle school I had my good friends around me, and I felt was treated no differently from oth-ers, everyone knew and accepted me even if we weren't in the same group. But I vividly remember my first day at senior school, which I was excitedly expecting to be the same (only better) and looking forward to the chance to make new friends. I walked into my class and everyone stopped talking, and then began sneaking looks and whispering to each other. That day no-one spoke to me, but I got stared at everywhere I went. By the end of the week I never wanted to go back to that school. ...'*
After talking it through with my parents, therapist, and the school, we agreed that I would do a presentation on my condition to the whole school. I was very scared, but I practised with my therapist and the principal sup-ported me by introducing me and talking a bit first. I felt amazed and proud of myself that I had the courage to do that, and I think it came in part from all the support I had experienced in my old school, as well as the help I had from people around me. Afterwards things completely changed because people understood why I looked different. It was tough, but now I've made friends again and I'm not afraid of school.

This is an account given by a young person with an established basis for self-confidence and good social skills. She had caring adults she could disclose her concerns to, so thankfully a pattern of school avoidance and refusal was prevented. Help needs to be offered in a timely way in these circumstances, which means that schools and parents need access to good services.

In the UK there is currently only one NHS outpatient service providing support for people with appearance concerns, based in the North Bristol Trust. The service bases its interventions on social skills training and CBT therapy, with research evidence to support effectiveness (Kleve et al. 2002).

Transition groups are offered for children about to move to secondary school with the aim of helping them manage teasing, develop assertiveness and role play friendship skills (Maddern et al. 2006). If it is likely this will be needed an early referral is best, as timing really matters. Alternatively (as mentioned before), other opportunities and online support can be found from specialist support groups and charities like CLAPA and Changing Faces. These are valuable resources, but accessed by a relatively small number of people, compared with the numbers who are affected. The confidence to take up these training opportunities may already have been impaired, or concerned adults may simply be unaware they are available.

> If the young person has had a difficult start in a new school, they may already have stopped attending, which makes re-introducing them more difficult. These resources can be used in individual therapy as an aid to recovery, but a team approach may be more effective for school re-entry.

When Love Beckons (or Not)

Even for resilient young people intentions can be hard to read, and this can be an incentive to avoid taking a chance on romance. One young woman interviewee described such an occasion at secondary school. Two boys in her subject class (where she excelled) were always teasing which made her uncomfortable, though over time she learned how to handle them. Later, as they approached GCSE time one of them asked her out. Though she was pleased to be asked, she was uncertain how to respond because of their previous (fairly recent) behaviour. Having thought about it, she declined. Later she heard them laughing about it, so she concluded that asking her out was a 'dare'. But even if he really liked her, at this age he might have coped with a rejection by shaming her in an immature way. It is possible that he may not have been entirely certain what his real intentions were, and ridicule is a ready defence if someone looks a bit different. She still isn't sure, and this is currently impacting her decisions about romantic relationships.

> How would you have advised her to deal with or interpret this situation?

It is often the case that young people who have already experienced teasing or bullying in relation to their appearance begin to withdraw, understandably anticipating negative responses from others, which in turn limits their opportunity for new and different encounters. This is equally true for those who are not visibly different but have been singled out for some other reason. Withdrawal limits their experience of themselves in relation to others, so their fears are not tested, or abilities developed. For others around them, understanding how to recognise and talk about avoidance and help them cope in the best way can be complicated. It is important to respect the person's right to develop at their own pace, tread water for a while and change their minds without loss of face. For example, someone may be choosing to identify as asexual because that is the truth for them, or it may be a cool way of saying 'I'm not ready to deal with this'. Neither is necessarily a problem if they have an active social life and interests which help them build confidence in themselves.

A pattern of avoidance in several areas, linked with low self-esteem, is a sign that they are uncertain how to take the next step forward in their lives or possibly what it might be. A supportive group is an antidote, but one to one therapy which does not end before those contacts are established may be needed first. At this point they may be very resistant to the idea of going to a group, never a popular choice for people struggling with mental health issues. Both children and young people are also sensitive to interventions that make them stand out from their peers, so will vary in their readiness and ability to speak about differences, at every stage (O'Dell and Prior 2004).

The mentalisation-based approach to integrative treatment is particularly helpful to practitioners wanting to reflect on how their well-intended interventions are actually experienced by young people. It seeks to support curiosity in therapists who may be struggling to reach out to their young clients. For instance, this group may see a 'straight talking' therapist approach as stigmatising and shaming if they often experience fear and shame. Similarly, an interested, committed, therapist stance may be perceived as patronising and intrusive. What the therapist hopes is 'authentic and boundaried' or 'holding hope' may not be communicating, and an angry or disinterested response from the client can quickly undermine the work if it is not understood and worked through. Blaming the client is not unheard of! For more resources on this issue, see manuals.annafreud.org/ambit/index.

Part 2: The Democratisation of Media, and the Construction of Difference in the Modern Age

Much has changed since Goffman's analysis of stigma, though recent research found empirical support for his categories of 'the own, and the wise (re-named as supporters, and stigmatisers') (Smith 2012). A person's identity can project itself into the virtual world, potentially increasing the possibilities for self-representation, though not always acceptance.

The World Is Smaller and Much Bigger

During adolescence and young adulthood sensitivities and anxieties increase for many young people, and the challenges of negotiating romantic relationships, going to college or entering the workplace require an established level of resilience and self-belief. The rise of social media has complicated the transition to young adulthood, with little space left for private mistakes that are not preserved forever in cyberspace. Online gaming does potentially offer opportunities to play with others, creating an 'avatar' which can offer a precious experience of being 'just like everyone else' and sometimes close online friendships for those with disabilities. A very moving example of this is the story of a young Norwegian man called Mats who died of Duchenne Muscular Dystrophy in 2014. His parents thought he had a very sad, limited life as his disease took hold, but were very surprised to discover that he was known all over Europe as Lord Ibelin Redmoor, nobleman, detective and philanderer in Azeroth. Friends came to his funeral and told of his online life and loves, which had extended beyond the game world with some people. He wrote *'in this world a girl wouldn't see a wheelchair or anything different. They would get my heart, soul and mind conveniently placed in a handsome, strong body. Luckily, pretty much every character in this virtual world looks great'* (Vicky Schaubert for BBC online February 2019, first published by NRK, Norway).

What do you know about your client's life in virtual worlds? Do you think it is relevant, helpful, or part of the problem? How might you find out more?

Avatars can offer relief and the experience of freedom, but for those with physical freedom too much online time can delay the development of real-world experience. Also, there are commercial pressures as equipment and accessories must be bought. Teenagers and young people are 'a market', and the images presented to them are often of conventionally attractive models and musicians, used to market the clothes, music and experiences that identify different transient tribes like 'cybergoths' or 'steampunk', 'emo', 'normcore', 'sneakerhead', 'yuccie' (in 2018 reportedly young creative individuals who wear olive green, black and grey!) and so on. This form of social signalling can be helpful, as anyone can take part if they wear the right clothes and makeup, and like the right bands. But it does take motivation and a thick skin to keep 'putting yourself out there' in the real world when your face or body doesn't fit the stereotype.

Life in the Pre-digital Age

People with visible difference who grew up before the 1990s, (when psychologists were first included as part of surgical teams) may have not met many, or any others with experiences like their own, where now there are many ways to connect with similar others online. For the most part, they had to work out issues on their own, or with the help of family and friends. This was a big disadvantage, and increased feelings of isolation and difference. But the upside of this earlier period was that people were more likely to meet for the first time and get to know each other face to face, rather than behind a screen, and they did not have to create a 'profile' to do it. So, the dilemma of 'when do I mention difference' did not arise.

> Have you written an online profile yourself? Did you find it easy, or difficult? How might that process have been different if you had a visible difference? What do you think the concerns are for someone now in their 50s who joins an online dating site for the first time? How would you talk about this with a client?

This young man describes his experience when he was still awaiting some appearance altering surgery in the pre-digital age.

'*it wasn't until my teenage years that the leg pulling started. I'd get a few stares having a drink in the bar. But then I looked bloody ugly to be honest. I was very self-conscious. If anyone even mentioned my cleft I'd scarper. I was painfully shy with girls too, although I had a couple of girlfriends. They must have been brave because they'd get a lot of comments like, 'Couldn't you do better than that?'* (Sunday Express, February 2nd 2014). Clearly the girls thought he was worth it though.

Sometimes romance can seem just too risky, so people accept being 'friend-zoned', and never tell someone they are really attracted to how they feel. *'In my late teens and early 20s I was very self-conscious about being rejected and thought I couldn't have relationships in the same way as my friends because I might not be that attractive to the opposite sex. I did get very low at this time, because I thought "well no-one will want me"* (man in his 50s quoted in Stock et al. 2015).

Moving Away for the First Time

For most, college or university are a time to expand social horizons and maybe meet someone they want to be closer to. Moving away to live and study is an important milestone, but even those who have been confident social actors at school and among their home friends can find it hard. Some may have extra support from a disability volunteer to help them get to lectures and events, and a caring, friendly relationship can be a great boost. Students volunteer for these roles and they can be of social benefit to both parties. However, the kindness and care can be misconstrued, and romantic hopes aroused. When they pluck up the courage to say how they are starting to feel it can come as a great shock to be told that their helper, who they had come to think of as a friend could never think of them 'in that way'. As Liz Carr the actor comments '*many people use the right "language" but they still see me as a cripple, if you see what I mean. So they use the proper term, but they still look at me and say "Yeah, but I wouldn't want to sleep with her"*' (from an interview by Mary O'Hara, Weds 21 June 2006, Guardian).

While the occasional 'fail' is part of 'normal' experience for people, it is never nice, and has a devastating edge for someone genuinely uncertain if

> Part of maturing is coming to terms with the fact that not everyone you are attracted to will feel the same way about you. That is different from feeling that you have been labelled 'undateable' though. What are the similarities and differences between this and being 'friend-zoned'. How might you help a client struggling with this?

they are acceptable. It can feel painful for the person turning them down too, who may feel that they have done something wrong. They may *have* committed the mistake of careless language, but the reaction to the hurt can seem extreme to them. A similar situation is explored in the film 'Wonder' where Augie comes to school at Halloween disguised in a costume, one of the rare days he can feel like everyone else. He overhears a boy he thinks of as his best friend make a cruel comment about him in order to appease a group of boys who bully him. The friendship and Augie's confidence are shattered, though it is made clear later that his friend really regrets it.

Young people report that the digital world is a mixed blessing at best, (while it is hard to imagine life without it) and the permanence of every photo, comment and blog in cyberspace can be a real problem when someone makes a mis-step while trying to work out who they are. We are more aware than ever about the impact of cyber bullying, but it is often hidden from family and friends.

> How might you encourage a young client to open up about these issues? What strategies might you suggest? Does an age difference between you and your client make this more difficult, or not. Would you ask?

In the arena of romance, 'friends with benefits', or 'hookups' there are many occasions for this kind of unintended pain, and the fears it activates. For this reason, many young people with visible differences are slower to begin dating in the digital age, which appears to be made more difficult by the increased use of media and online platforms to meet people. As one young woman comments *'whenever I meet someone who has met their partner in real life rather than online, I'm like "How? What magic did you do?"'* (Fox-Leonard 2018). While a 2018 Changing Faces survey showed that only 33% had used a dating app, 90% of those with visible difference had received negative comments or feedback. '*When I was 18, I met all the people I dated in bars, but now the only way you can meet someone romantically is through an app. And it just feels so much scarier that way, because it feels like you've got even more to hide*' (Boudicca Fox-Leonard, Daily Telegraph 17 Nov 2018).

According to Changing Faces six in ten respondents to their survey had avoided going on dates because of their appearance. The issue of 'when to tell' about a difference is a live one, and then if things don't work out, it is very easy to read too much into other people's awkwardness. Online dating is still stigmatised in some contexts, but many more people do it. For everyone, lots of choice makes it hard to choose, and it is easy to pursue the fantasy that there is another, better option out there maybe just a swipe away.

People with visible differences experience fewer online responses, more weird questions and 'ghosting' (when the other person suddenly stops responding). At the same time adults without disabilities most commonly misrepresent themselves on dating sites in relation to physical appearance, especially weight, age and height. If the difference is not visible in a photo, should you tell or not? Most would like to get this issue out of the way, but how it is broached can make a big difference.

> One interviewee in her 40s who had 2 episodes of online dating reported that after a period of awkward meetings she decided it was best to 'skype' or 'Facetime' before the standard 'coffee' meeting, to see the other persons reactions, and so they could see her. What other strategies might be helpful?

Learning from Normal Disappointments

With or without a difference it is a tough environment online, and many people who consider themselves 'normal' find it very demoralising, especially if they are not young and good looking. Articles which talk about setbacks of the dating experience can help to put these experiences into context. A positive mental attitude and resilience are needed, for instance 'it's a great way to meet interesting people' or 'it helps to learn how to talk to strangers', but this is more easily achieved if your worth as a human being is not felt to be at stake.

Others have developed the view that their difference/disability is a 'filter' which acts as a natural barrier to sift out people who wouldn't be right for them, which is a more helpful approach, though not always true. What matters is to find a way to talk about it, without making it more significant than it needs to be and creating a space to find out more about the other person's strengths and fears. This does require a level of perceptiveness about character that takes experience to acquire.

And Hard-Won Lessons

Boudicca Fox-Leonard reports (*Telegraph* 17/11/18) that for one young woman, the turning point in her love life was when she stopped feeling like she had a secret to tell '*for a long time I felt like I was obligated to tell people that I had scars, like I needed to tell them that I was damaged goods. Often the first thing dates knew about me was my illness and the scars. My whole identity was wrapped up around them*' as a result her relationships were often unhealthy too '*I'd put up with treatment that wasn't OK because I felt like I was lucky that someone was deigning to be with me, despite all my flaws*'. After getting help, her advice to others with visible differences is '*Just because you have a scar or physical difference, doesn't mean you owe people your story. If someone likes you, they should like you for yourself.*'

This strength is something to take pride in, but it is also good to be generous with other people's weaknesses, if you can. If they are in the 'normal' range but lack confidence themselves, they may find it hard to be alongside someone who looks different, and they have not had a lifetime to learn how to deal with it. As one interviewee, reflecting back on her dating experiences in the 1970s and 1980s commented '*I was always afraid that they would leave me, and I put too much pressure on my first relationships by being clingy and suspicious of their other friendships with women. It must have been very difficult for them, and I can see now that I spoiled some promising beginnings by not being independent enough.*'

Someone who is different must also be careful not to internalise stigma and become overly suspicious of 'normals' who want a relationship with a different or disabled person. They will have their own reasons, and it helps to understand what they are. Commenting on her own development another interviewee said '*I used to think inner beauty was a load of rubbish, but now I don't. … After dating this really good-looking man for a while I felt so relaxed with him, and I asked him if he noticed my difference right away, he said yes (to my surprise as there was no negative reaction). When I asked him what he thought about it he said "I liked the way you looked and thought you must be an interesting person because of the experiences you have had, more than an average pretty face. It showed in the way you were with other people".*

This comment comes from a mature and insightful woman. It is interesting to note that she was not sure her boyfriend had noticed her difference. If it is never mentioned people with visible differences can be left wondering if the other is just very unobservant! Better to find a way to make a non-stigmatising reference, anecdote or sincere compliment.

A therapist working with someone who is visibly different needs to ask in what way our increasingly secular and commercial worldview makes a difference to their client's valuing of self. Their age and interests will impact on their experience of difference in complex ways. The age of robotics, identity politics, social media and cosmetic surgery is altering how we construct ourselves, both in our own minds and in the world. Though this scope is huge, it is important to hold in mind the relevance, usefulness and difficulties of these issues to the individual and the therapy context. The effort to assert an identity not focused on physical appearance in the twenty-first century is both more complex and necessary. The person in front of the therapist, or indeed behind their PC screen, may have a complex online identity, which enhances, or perhaps replaces much of their face-to-face life if they are avoidant. It is important for the therapist to ask themselves and their client questions about their significance and relevance to the therapeutic conversation.

What do you mean when you talk about your 'self', and what does your client mean? Is this a necessary question?

References

Bonnano A, Choi JY, (2010) Mapping out the social experience of cancer patients with facial disfigurement. Health 2(5).

Bradbury E (1997) Understanding the problems. In: Lansdown R, Rumsey N, Bradbury E, Carr T, Partridge J (eds) Visibly different: coping with disfigurement. Reed Educational and Professional Publishing Ltd, Oxford.

Burke S (2020) Break the Mould: How to take your place in the World. Published by Wren and Rook UK

Changing Faces (2010) Teaching resources available from http://www.changing-faces.org.uk/Education/Teaching-resources

Cline T, Proto A, Raval P, Paolo TD (1998) The effects of brief exposure and of classroom teaching on attitudes children express towards facial disfigurement in peers. Educational Research 40:55–68

Department for Education (2014) Early education and childcare. http://www.assets.publishing.service.gov.uk

Kish V, Lansdown R (2000) Meeting the psychosocial impact of facial disfigurement: developing a clinical service for children and families. Clinical Child Psychology and Psychiatry 5(4):497–512

Kleve L, Rumsey N, Wyn-Williams M, White P (2002) The effectiveness of cognitive-behavioural interventions provided at Outlook: a disfigurement support unit. Journal of Evaluation in Clinical Practice 8(4):387–395

Lansdown R, Rumsey N, Bradbury E, Carr T, Partridge J (1997) Visibly different: Coping with disfigurement. Reed Educational and Professional Publishing Ltd.

Maddern LH, Cadogan JC and Emerson MP (2006) 'Outlook' A psychological service for children with a different appearance. Clinical Child Psychology and Psychiatry 11(3):431–433

O'Connor A (2018) Practice guide: equality and diversity. Nursery World (online magazine). Published by MA Education, London.

O'Dell L, Prior J, (2004) Evaluating a schools service for children with facial disfigurement: the views of teaching and support staff. Support for Learning. 20(1):2–47. Wiley Blackwell.

Palacio RJ (2012) Wonder. Corgi Books, London.

Smith R (2012) Segmenting an audience into the own, the wise and Normals: a latent class analysis of stigma-related categories. Communications Research Reports (29ed) 29(4): 257–265.

Stock NM, Whale K (2011) An evaluation of a school-based intervention to promote positive attitudes and behaviours towards people with facial disfigurement: Main study report. Centre for Appearance Research, Bristol.

Stock NM, Billaud Feragen K, Rumsey N, (2015) 'It doesn't all stop at 18' psychological adjustment and support needs of adults born with a cleft lip and/or palate. The Cleft Palate-Craniofacial Journal 52(5):543–554

Vannatta K, Gartstein MA, Zeller M, Noll RB, (2009) Peer acceptance and social behaviour during childhood and adolescence: how important are appearance, athleticism, and academic competence? International Journal of Behavioural Development 33(4):303–311

6

Assessment and Treatment Planning

This section will offer practical guidance on assessment and the development of an integrative treatment plan, with suggestions on using resources from Acceptance and Commitment (ACT), Mentalisation and Compassion Focused therapy as well as CBT where needed. A few examples of presentations and treatment plans will be given to illustrate, but these are intended to be food for thought rather than the only 'right' approach. In most a different model could be used if it is a better 'fit' with the client, with the assumption that treatment includes an explicit method of identifying suitable goals and assessing outcomes. Your client may first present with appearance concerns, or these could be a 'background' issue they have made adjustments to which are un-necessarily limiting now.

© The Author(s) 2020
V. Purcell, *Understanding Visible Differences*, Palgrave Texts in Counselling and Psychotherapy, https://doi.org/10.1007/978-3-030-51655-0_6

Working with a Stepped Approach to Appearance Issues

The PLISSIT (Permission, Limited Information, Specific Suggestions, Intensive Treatment, Clarke et al. 2014) acronym stands for a framework of stepped care intended to promote psychosocial adjustment in appearance, which many working in the NHS or similar situations will find a familiar concept. It is an additional resource for thinking about the structure of treatment planning, while retaining some flexibility of therapeutic approach.

Level one of this model concerns obtaining permission to talk about the person's appearance, and a sensitive exploration of psychosocial concerns. This level of conversation is conducted by GPs, practice nurses, Psychological Wellbeing Practitioners and professional health care helplines, which may be done prior to referral for further treatment. Some of these contacts are not face to face, so unless the person raises appearance as a concern it may not be included in referral information.

Level two involves limited information giving by health practitioners including doctors and nurses working with target groups. This includes written leaflets, support group and website information, as well as giving basic information about visible difference to (for example) those recovering from disfiguring surgery, or new parents.

Level three includes the giving of specific advice or interventions for 'target stressors', like social skills training, help on dealing with staring and comments as well as how to manage social situations. Professionals at this level are trained in the relevant skills and work with access to supervision. Clinical nurse specialists, occupational therapists, maxillofacial technicians and some members of specialist support groups are in this category.

At Level four more intensive treatments are offered with the aim of improving functioning and modifying 'maladaptive appearance schemas'. Clinicians identified as suitable (in the Clarke 2014 model) include clinical psychologists and CBT therapists, where the client has a mood disorder and multiple appearance related concerns, shame proneness, reassurance seeking, avoidance and checking which are not recent in origin.

What Difference Does It Make If You Work in a General Mental Health Setting?

The guidelines above were designed with specialist services in mind. However, as previously noted many clients will present to a general adult mental health service or private practitioner, who must assess whether they have the skills and supervision necessary to help effectively.

Therapists need to be aware of the complexity of their interaction with a client who may have suffered as a result of social stigma and be sensitive to shame triggers. Most clinicians would agree that commenting on appearance, for instance saying 'it doesn't look that bad' or minimising the importance of appearance are very unlikely to help the patient believe that the therapist has understood. If the clinician's own appearance is in the normal range this is particularly true, and the client may experience it as alienating, or even conclude that the therapist is unlikely to be helpful. Later in treatment, work to adjust the importance placed on physical appearance may become central, but first the client should believe that the clinician has understood what it is like to be the subject of staring, comments and negative stereotyping. If the therapist is new to this type of encounter a review of the 'Tyrion' character in 'Game of Thrones' might help to inform them about the common experiences, sensitivities, humour and strengths developed by this way of living. Most importantly, to note that the significant contribution the character makes in his (fictional) world, his concerns, and interests have nothing to do with his difference. For him it is something that gets in the way in other people's minds, which can occasionally blindside him.

Talking About Difference

If the clinician is working alongside a surgical or outpatient team raising the subject of the client's visible difference where needed will probably be straightforward, as it is the focus of the clinic. Even those who are very sensitive about questioning in this area report feeling less so in this context, as they expect more expertise and a better understanding. It can be more complicated in a student or general adult mental health setting.

Ideally during the assessment process the therapist and patient will consider briefly how appearance concerns intersect with other presenting problems, as part of agreeing the treatment plan. But if some aspects are hard to approach, the most important thing is to note that there is an issue which may emerge later in treatment, and ensure that the interpersonal groundwork is laid, so that when the client is able to (or feels it is necessary to) speak, it can be done in a congruent way. Often asking about whether the client was bullied at school during the routine assessment is enough to raise the subject. Most will have been to some extent, at some time.

Their response to this question can then guide you about where to go next—you need to understand more about their relationship with themselves, and how both bullying and growing up in an environment of beauty bias might have impacted on that. Do they sometimes have a cruel, punishing or hopeless relationship with their vulnerable self for instance, and how does that interact with their presenting problem? Or do they have assumptions about the unspoken prejudice of others with 'normal' appearance which might impact your therapeutic alliance? The therapist also needs to have a working understanding of their medical treatment 'journey', which will require a few careful questions, and some independent research rather than a lengthy inquisition.

Objectification Theory (Frederickson and Roberts 1997) and related work can be helpful frameworks for thinking about how repeated experiences of social exclusion, bullying or stigmatisation can lead to the development of specific appearance concerns, presenting as similar to those in social anxiety. Focusing particularly on women, it describes how the body becomes separated from personal identity, '*as if the body/body parts are capable of representing her'* (Augustus-Horvath and Tylka 2009) and the person is socialised to internalise an observer's perspective as their primary view of their physical selves. This leads to a habitual monitoring of outward appearances, linked with feelings of anxiety, shame and disgust towards the self, potentially disconnecting from internal states. Researchers have also noted an inhibition in social situations, obstructing peak motivational states which require a 'forgetting' of the external appearance.

Alternatively, depending on the support they have received from family and school some people will have built up good interpersonal skills and healthy defences as a result of earlier difficulties. Noting these strengths and including them as resources in the formulation will contribute to building the working alliance. Checking whether the client has found it necessary to cope by using avoidance strategies which limit their lives now, and the difficulties which caused this needs to be approached in an empathic way. A timeline and functional analysis are useful tools to 'map' these experiences and choices, noting what might have been missed as a result. This can help when thinking about the inclusion of values work or a compassion focus in the treatment plan.

Assessing the Impact of Internalised Shame and External Sources of Shame

If earlier abuse and trauma has been severe and your client lacked support, they may have internalised a negative and destructive attitude to themselves at a time when they were too young to understand or process experiences. Often when able to recount these experiences of abuse they are told in a vivid way, with word-for-word descriptions. In this case it is wise to assess for other indicators of trauma and whether they need to be worked with as a priority.

Here we should note that shame is a common experience, though intensely painful. As Lewis (2003) comments '*while primary emotions require a self to experience the state, self-conscious emotions require a self both to produce the state and then to experience it. For instance, a loud noise may put me into a state of fright. But to experience this I need to be aware of my state of fright. To be in a state of shame I need to compare my action against some standard, either my own or someone else's. My failure, relative to the standard, results in a state of shame.'*

Shame is a moral or social emotion which can be internal or external and arises through self-reflection. For instance, someone who abuses another person may acknowledge that others will disapprove of their actions. If they have contravened their own internalised moral code they will feel ashamed of themselves. On the other hand, if they feel that despite this social judgement they are entitled to behave as they did because of their beliefs, this shame will be external, simply an awareness of the disapproval of others, something to be avoided without self-judgement.

It is also important to make the distinction between shame and guilt clear. Guilt arises from negative evaluation of a specific behaviour which is perceived as chosen in some way. It may be associated with shame for the act, having failed to meet one's own standards, but it is possible at least theoretically to apologise, make amends and be forgiven. People who are bullied for looking different are basically being shamed for existing and are not able to escape it, though other aspects of behaviour may also be included in the abuse (like shyness, the way they move, or eat). Where the abused person lacks caring support their sense of their own value will be negatively affected.

'**Toxic shame**' (Tomkins 1963) is the phrase sometimes used for pervasive internalised shame—where the person feels that they are unloveable, unacceptable in a way that they are unable to repair because it is a social judgement. It is not necessarily related to appearance and may have arisen due to inescapable circumstances which were not really understood—for example children may feel responsible for their parent's divorce. Such an association will remain until it is brought to awareness and challenged. However, this intensity of feeling tends to be repressed and is often not easily offered as a disclosure even in a helpful therapeutic situation. A 'third person' discussion, for instance the therapist saying something like 'in my experience people who have been bullied often experience a sense of shame, even though there is no reason to' can create the space to refer to these feelings without being overwhelmed by them. Toxic shame can sometimes develop following sexual or physical abuse in young children, occurring at a time when the brain is both immature and being shaped by experience, where there are many experiences of shame-inducing negative feedback and little or no unconditional positive regard.

A person who feels shame as a result of a failure to meet socially sanctioned appearance standards may also experience regret (for being the way they are), and alienation from the aspect of themselves which has been shamed (*I hate my birthmark*!). It is associated with embarrassment, a self-conscious emotion, which raises blood pressure and heart rate, though this normally arises in a social context. An important distinction between embarrassment and shame is that if someone makes an embarrassing mistake, they may be able to laugh about it later (think of slipping on a banana skin). People who are shamed and see themselves as vulnerable to shaming are unable to separate from a behaviour act/thought (they are just being), what shames them is regarded as a judgement on self. But again, don't assume this is the case. The person in front of you may have a robust and healthy narcissism, and want help figuring out how to deal with an image-obsessed, prejudiced world and stay sane. One thought experiment which can help is to imagine yourself living your client's life for a time, with their appearance, experiences and personality. How would you do?

Sadly, in many cultures shaming women (particularly) over appearance is a common behaviour, to the extent that even beautiful young women fear it and spend much time and money trying to avoid it. Media and commercial interests exploit these anxieties and shockingly, in 2019 teenagers are requesting lip fillers for Christmas presents as face and body 'sculpting' becomes normalised by shows like 'Love Island'. Appearance anxiety may be triggered by an unguarded comment from a parent, friend or romantic interest and is a common therapy presentation in adolescents and young people. The longing to always be the most beautiful/desirable young person in the room may seem narcissistic and insecure, but safety in avoiding shame is often the underlying motivation. Increasing numbers of young men also feel the pressure to seek the perfect body by using steroids and exercise, leading to a newly appreciated disorder—'Bigorexia' where exercise and steroids are abused to achieve an unrealistic image. Young people who experience peer victimisation are at greater risk of developing mental health problems, and Irwin et al. (2016) report that body shame is an underlying emotional mechanism, resulting in social anxiety for girls and higher levels of externalising problems in boys.

The term external shame (which often drives problems like bigorexia) refers to the distressing awareness that others view the self negatively (Gilbert and Andrews 1998; Gilbert and Miles 2002). Gilbert comments *'much social behaviour is about attempts to control social interactions (to maximise benefits and minimise harms), it is our ability to have models of ourselves as we exist in the minds of others that is often the key to human social interaction. We need to know if we are attractive to others or not.'* Attractiveness is at least partly a performance, and it is quite easy to get this social assessment wrong. We are familiar with performances which fail—the stereotypes are the raw material of comedy, but there can be ambiguity in our view of ourselves, or it may be situation-specific. A woman may correctly assess that she is attractive with her 'face on' (make up) but believe that she isn't without it.

An anxious awareness that others may be evaluating appearance negatively can result in an over-reaction to a thoughtless or mis-heard comment, and clinicians working with Body Dysmorphic Disorder often learn that the problem was triggered by something similar. Patterns of rumination and selective attention magnify and maintain the concern (Clarke et al. 2009), to the extent that in extreme cases the person may regard themselves as completely unacceptable to others in a social context and stop going out.

As Gilbert goes on to point out, our evolved 'theory of mind', concerning what others think of us, is a source of shame if we believe or become aware that their judgement is negative. Anxieties may be aggravated by uncertainty about what people really think if there is a suspicion that they are 'just being nice' in the comments they make. A person may say 'I don't want to be seen like this', referring to a class of negative, shaming responses that they think will occur in the mind of the other (which they might not agree with). Crucially they believe it will lead to diminishment socially, devaluation, loss of power or rejection.

Or as we have noted in the case of burn victims they may say 'I can't be this person', a comment induced by their own inescapable judgement of their changed appearance (according to learned values) and fear of the judgement of others. This judgement of the self is internal shame, which can develop alongside (for instance) a child's theory of mind if they are not offered alternative ways of interpreting their experiences. In his analysis of the literature about the development of this capacity Gilbert and Miles (2002) comments '*presumably for people to internalise stigma they must see the other as having, if not the right, then the skill or power to judge them so. ... However, the moment a person refuses to accept the legitimacy of the "judger" or "rejecter" then they are also refusing to internalise*' (Camp et al. 2002). The burns survivor needs to adjust their own beliefs about the meaning of their own and other's appearance as part of building resilience, in order to manage their changed status in the minds of others.

Stigma consciousness refers to the awareness or feeling that one belongs to a category or class of person that is seen as having stigmatised traits, in this case appearance, though other attributes (like lower intelligence) might also be incorrectly associated.

The person who is born or becomes visibly different needs to have or develop additional skills in the performative aspect of social interactions, to ensure that they do not accept the stigmatising, or uninformed judgement of others, preferably in a polite and dignified way. For this reason, training to increase their range of social strategies may form part of the treatment plan, to help the client manage the discourse in awkward situations (rather than avoid them pre-emptively) and not agree to feel ashamed.

Questions which might help to tease these issues out:

(adapted from Rolland 2018)

Are there issues related to your difference that you think about to yourself but do not discuss openly?

What issues? Why do you keep them to yourself?

Under what circumstances would you discuss these private thoughts?

With whom would you feel most and least comfortable talking about these issues? Why?

Establishing a Therapeutic Relationship

Some experienced therapists suggest that the therapy process begins when therapist and client agree to meet, but the time between agreeing the date and before the actual or virtual meeting is often overlooked. An over-busy schedule allows less scope for both reflection and adaptation on both sides. Though this is improving, a clinic may not routinely let the client know what to expect in the first meeting, and if the person has had previous therapy this experience can strongly shape their expectations for better or worse. A phone call is a brief and useful 'bridge' worth considering, as it conveys more information and 'real experience' than a written exchange.

Within the constraints of their clinical culture it is the therapist's first job to **welcome the client**, put them at ease and inform them of the purpose of assessment. Finding out what brought them to treatment at this moment, and their hopes and fears in relation to therapy are an important part of that process, whether or not there are referral notes. Setting a collaborative tone means that assessment tasks should not dominate the experience of being met, while ensuring that the formal or informal agenda is attended to, and plans made for any activities prior to the next meeting.

In the early meetings the aim is to **establish a working relationship**, while doing a thorough assessment, and jointly develop a working case formulation to guide initial treatment planning, so that consent to treatment can be given. It is important to first understand what the immediate problems are, which will meet the client's expectation of focus, for instance if the person is highly anxious, what is happening, or not, in the everyday. In some detail. This leads easily on to developing an understanding of how things would be different if this was not a problem. The setting of clear and attainable goals, which are congruent with the person's values, is the basis for the perception of an (eventually) successful treatment episode and a strong working alliance. This is increasingly important if the therapist works in the 'payment by results' culture of the modern NHS, but in clinics where CBT is the dominant model it can lead inexperienced therapists to set goals which are relatively concrete and easy to achieve, but less relevant for the client. Where shame may be activated it can take time to discover what really matters. Remember to check if something important has been overlooked!

Your 'Therapeutic Stance': What Do Different Models Have to Say?

This is a complex topic, and as a qualified therapist you will have read, discussed and reflected deeply on it. To understand the thoughts, feelings and behaviours of another person is a challenge which requires intense focus. To add to the complexity, you have very limited time and a constrained context. This process can be difficult on both sides, because it sometimes evokes avoidant responses, unchallenged assumptions and even prejudice. Working through these leads to a genuine growth experience, though good supervision is often needed to reflect on and unpick events in the therapy room.

Bordin (1979) was the first to define three different aspects of the therapeutic relationship—the relational bond, the tasks of the therapy, and the therapeutic goals. The boom in research that followed this has firmly established the robust association between a good therapeutic alliance and successful outcomes across therapeutic models (Horvath and Bedi 2002). Therapists have a tendency to over-estimate how good their alliance with the client is.

While this is not a major topic in some training programmes researchers now broadly agree that the therapeutic alliance is a key factor in a good outcome, though in a meta-analysis Baldwin et al. (2007) found that the therapist's alliance was more predictive than the patients. Each of the major therapeutic models has something to say about the therapeutic relationship, or stance. While the identified tasks in therapy may guide therapist and client towards a particular change model, the rich interpersonal exchanges in the therapy setting benefit from sensitive and informed consideration, which has taken into account multiple factors. We all have our preferred or habitual ways of working. Below is a very brief summary of relevant therapeutic stances, some of which will be very familiar, others perhaps less so, to guide your curiosity.

A Systemic and/or Mentalising Approach

When working with a client who is visibly different a 'not-knowing' and open stance, avoiding any 'expert' therapeutic values, will help to create the space to discover how things are and what needs to change. Escudero (2016) in a discussion on systemic therapeutic alliances describes this stance as 'necessary but not sufficient' as part of the process of system mapping to generate and test hypotheses. As discussed in previous chapters, viewing the presenting issue in the context of multiple systems of meaning, many of which are not in the control of the client, can be helpful to both therapist and client. For example, what is the impact of an almost total absence of media images of women with facial differences? Is this greater for ethnic minority girls, and if so, in what ways? Do recent improvements in representation create new possibility fields? How are things different for young men, or older men?

Bronfenbrenner's (1992) ecological systems theory of child development imagines these systems as concentric circles: the 'macrosystem'—including economic, political, cultural, social and national constructs; the 'exosystem'—covering community, school, mass media and health agencies; and the 'microsystem'—closest to the person, family, peers, school/work and religion. Finally, the individual, who absorbs and interprets all these systems, thinking and acting in response to them. Denial may be an important, if temporary, defence—'it doesn't bother me!' against ideas and attitudes that may feel very threatening. Hopelessness, despair or anger may be managed in this way. As one interviewee said '*if you had asked me directly about my difference when I was younger, I would have fallen through the floor!*' In a worst-case scenario this denial is mirrored by the therapist, who feels disempowered and uncertain how to raise things which feel important.

For both, aspects of the mentalisation approach can serve to unblock communication. This model was developed to enhance the ability to understand what is in the mind of the other, and emotionally self-regulate, initially for clients with borderline personality disorders. Without this understanding interactions can sometimes be experienced as confusing or overwhelming. The therapist aims to develop a relationship in which the mental states of self and others can be explored, developing more rational representations of their thoughts and feelings. As in the systemic approach a curious, patient and questioning stance in exploration is used (Fonagy and Bateman 2006).

Systemic techniques of lineal and circular questioning can be used to elicit theories and ideas about the problem. Probes may generate further information, allowing the therapist to offer new ideas or descriptions, and contextualising makes connections between behaviour and patterns in the system. Therapist skills in 'matching' and reflecting back demonstrate empathy, and 'amplification' of a particular idea, affect, theme or behavioural sequence can explore its relevance and impact. In this approach an evolving formulation which may be revised later, is a process of discovery (Dallos and Draper 2015), to be tested with experience. While there are no detailed guidelines it is grounded by theoretical reference points, like attachment, power and gender. I would argue that whatever change model and techniques are used, the formulation of the problem and stance of the therapist benefits from consideration of the systemic perspective.

CBT and Third-Wave Therapies

Acceptance and Commitment (ACT)

As a third-wave cognitive behavioural model ACT seeks to promote flexible and voluntary contact with present values-based experiences, even difficult ones. It seeks to dissolve rigid and avoidant patterns which cause and maintain problems. Its basic stance is functional contextualism which de-emphasizes form over function (Vilardaga and Hayes 2009), meaning that any technique is merely a tool to achieve greater understanding, which could be substituted with another more relevant one as needed. The therapist stance is also flexible, using Relational Frame theory, and seeks to establish a necessary and sufficient relationship to achieve agreed, shared treatment goals.

To foster the relationship the therapist seeks to maintain an awareness of and connect with the experience of their client. While few therapists would disagree with this stance, specific techniques are used to bring this into focus in ACT. An example of this is the DEICTICS framing exercise which recommends taking a few minutes prior to a therapy session (Vilardaga et al. 2007). A form of immersive questioning and perspective taking is used to imaginatively enter the experience of their client coming to the session before returning to the therapist's own position. This deictic framing or perspective taking is at the core of ACT work along with an initial focus on values. Clearly defined goals and values are the core from which the therapeutic task is established. The therapeutic relationship must be robust enough to support the client in recognising that they are avoiding difficult things which really support their goals and values, and working to change these patterns of thought and behaviour.

Compassion Focused Therapy

The goal of this approach is for the client to achieve self-compassion. The therapist stance is supportive, demonstrating an attachment style which is stable and accepting. A compassionate interpretation of the client's experiences is modelled by the therapist, with the aim of developing capacities for self-soothing and affiliation to self in the client, reducing the threat response. At first this might be resisted by someone who is accustomed to a critical stance towards their own perceived shortcomings. For them, the value of this choice may lie in separation from aspects of self which are felt to be shameful or too painful. It is their 'socialised self' which stands in judgement on 'unreformable' difference. Often at this point the therapist will take a question to their supervisor, wondering if they have chosen the wrong model, when pacing is the problem. Referring to the systems of meaning may help put therapist and client in a sound alliance, as their new, more compassionate relationship with self will be forged in opposition to socially powerful narratives like 'beauty is best'.

Attributes of compassion are defined as sensitivity, sympathetic care for well-being, distress tolerance, non-judgement and empathy, and the therapist is expected to have the skill to deploy these as appropriate. Therapist's transformative skills include attention, use of imagery, reasoning, feeling, behaviour and sensory experiences (Gilbert 2009).

There is less written about the therapeutic relationship itself, but in common with all new wave therapies the stance is collaborative and supportive.

Cognitive Behavioural Stance

Although the therapeutic relationship was for many years not a training focus in CBT, one chapter of the original 'Bible' written by Aaron Beck— 'Cognitive Therapy of Depression' (1979) was devoted to the importance of a strong therapeutic alliance as an essential component of treatment. There Beck refers to the 'core conditions' of Carl Rogers' humanistic therapy—congruence, accurate empathy and unconditional positive regard as 'necessary but not sufficient', separating cognitive therapy from this approach. After this the therapeutic relationship received little focus in concentrated training programmes in the UK, but now there is a recognition and renewed interest in relationship factors that support collaboration, empiricism and socratic dialogue (Kazantzis et al. 2017).

Because CBT is a technical therapy, agreement on tasks and focus is considered the foundation of the therapeutic alliance, though some other models might regard this as putting the 'cart before the horse'. It is also the area where resistance is frequently encountered, leading to a recognition that some groups, particularly older adults and survivors of different types of abuse *'may require more attention to the emotional elements of the therapeutic relationship for effective therapy to take place'* (Lavender 2019).

'Collaborative empiricism' is considered central to the work, with a supportive and curious stance from the therapist to encourage the collection of data relevant to the issues in the patient's life. Data logs and mood diaries help to map the issues and formulate a plan for recovery primarily focused on problem resolution rather than insight (which would also be regarded as necessary but not sufficient!).

Some Considerations and Tools for Assessment

Additional measures which can help with assessment and treatment planning where there are appearance issues include the *Derriford Appearance* scale short form (Carr et al. 2000), which measures social anxiety and social avoidance, the *Physical Appearance Discrepancy* scale (Altable 1996) and the *Brief fear of Negative Evaluation* scale (Leary 1983). Recent research conducted by the Appearance Research Collaboration found that a dispositional bias towards optimism was associated with good adjustment, and the *Life Orientation Test Revised (LOT-R)* (Scheier and Carver 1987) was the measure they used to assess this. This does not mean that clients with a more pessimistic disposition cannot do well, but it helps to have identified this difference at the start of work.

Is Your Client a 'Customer for Change'?

In their seminal work on assessing readiness for change, Prochaska et al. (1992) identified five potential stages in the process of planning and implementing behaviour change. A good piece of therapeutic work will not rush the early stages and aims can still be discussed in the spirit of 'when you feel ready'.

The first stage is pre-contemplation, where the person is not intending to make changes in the next 6 months (sometimes characterized as 'resistant'). People in this stage find information helpful, particularly when it is related to the effects of not changing. Creating a timeline for change helps them to avoid remaining stuck and prepare to be ready. Prospective and retrospective work can still be helpful, but goal setting needs to reflect their current stance.

Contemplation refers to the position where there is an intention to change in the next 6 months, but the client is not ready for an action-oriented programme. Work on the pros and cons of change may be perceived as evenly balanced, but clients are very sensitive to the risks associated with change. Bear in mind that they may be correctly assessing the lack of time and resources to do more immediately.

In the third, preparation stage the client may already have a plan in mind, and typically will already have taken some significant action towards that (like coming to see a therapist for help in creating change.)

The person in the fourth 'action' stage has already made significant overt changes to aspects of their lifestyle and are in the process of moving towards achievement of their aims.

Finally, those in the maintenance stage have made the changes they want and are seeking ways to troubleshoot or prevent relapse. This stage is estimated to last between six months and five years. In each stage once you as therapist have understood what they want from sessions the stage is set for work to proceed more smoothly.

Consider what might be unspoken—Sometimes people present in therapy with one issue because the larger, buried one is too much to address at that particular moment. They may recognize that psychological change is needed, or alternatively, they may have been pursuing a medical intervention, hoping a difference could be 'fixed', and psychological treatment is recommended instead. They may need to talk through what that means for them, to ensure they really want to engage, rather than just attend to satisfy a surgeon's requirement so that they can access surgery. Reluctant patients can be the hardest ones to work with, as psychological solutions are seen as second best, or beside the point. However, there is useful work to do, which may encourage them to return to therapy post-surgery, when or if the hoped-for change in how they feel has not happened.

Talk about it—You may be wondering where your client is on this scale when you first meet them, and it is best to discuss it with them during the assessment process and ask them what they think. Asking your client to reflect on this could be an early between-session task. It is helpful in establishing a collaborative working alliance, and to dispel any fears they have about being pushed, feeling exposed, or having to promise to change in order to get help. Once you are both clear, you are ready to talk about the changes in their life they would like to see in more detail, whether this is a soon as possible, next year, or in five years' time.

Here the crucial questions are always a variant on 'when your life has changed in the ways that you want it to, how will you know?' To clarify, 'what will be different?' If the answer is a vague, 'I will be happier', then you need develop a detailed description of what that means, and again, how they will know.

The general advice that whatever goals are agreed should be SMART— Specific, Measurable, Achievable, Realistic and Timed—is useful in many approaches to treatment as it allows the therapist and client to assess their direction and progress at different stages in the work.

References

Altable M (1996) Issues in the assessment and treatment of body image disturbance in culturally diverse populations. In: Thompson JK (ed) Eating disorders, obesity and body image: a practical guide to assessment and treatment. American Psychological Association Books, Washington DC.

Augustus-Horvath CL, Tylka TL, (2009) A test and extension of objectification theory as it predicts disordered eating: does women's age matter? *Journal of Counselling Psychology* 56(2):253–265

Baldwin SA, Wampold BE, Imel ZE, (2007) Untangling the alliance-outcome correlation: exploring the relative importance of therapist and patient variability in the alliance. *Journal of Consulting and Clinical Psychology* 75:842–852

Beck A (1979) Cognitive therapy of depression. Guildford Press.

Bordin ES (1979) The generalizability of the psychoanalytic concept of the working alliance. Psychotherapy: Theory, research and practice 16:252–260.

Bronfenbrenner U (1992) Ecological systems theory. In: Vasta R (ed) Six theories of child development: revised formulations and current issues. Jessica Knightley Publishers, London, pp 187–249.

Camp DL, Finlay WML, Lyons E (2002) Is low self-esteem an inevitable consequence of stigma? An example from women with chronic mental health problems. *Social Science and Medicine* 55:823–824

Carr A, Moss T, Harris D, (2000) The Derriford appearance scale (DAS59): a new scale to measure individual responses to living with problems of appearance. *British Journal of Health Psychology* 5:201–215

Clarke A, Veale D, Wilson R (2009) Overcoming body image problems including body Dysmorphic disorder. Constable and Robinson Ltd, London.

Clarke A, Thompson AR, Jenkinson E, Rumsey N, Newell R (2014) CBT for appearance anxiety: psychosocial interventions for anxiety due to visible difference. Wiley Blackwell.

Dallos R, Draper R (2015) An introduction to theory and practice, 4th edn. Open University Press, McGraw Hill Education, Berkshire.

Escudero V (2016) Guest editorial: the therapeutic alliance from a systemic perspective [Editorial]. Journal of Family Therapy 38(1):1–4

Fonagy P, Bateman AW (2006) Mechanisms of change in mentalisation-based treatment of BPD. Journal of Clinical Psychology 62(4):411–430

Frederickson BL, Roberts TA (1997) Objectification Theory: Towards understanding women's lived experiences and mental health risks. *Psychology of women quarterly* 21:173–206

Gilbert P (2009) Introducing compassion-focused therapy. Advances in Psychiatric Treatment 15:199–208

Gilbert P, Andrews B (eds) (1998) Shame: interpersonal behavior, psychopathology and culture. Oxford University Press, New York.

Gilbert P, Miles J (eds) (2002) Body shame: conceptualisation, research and treatment. Routledge, London.

Horvath AO, Bedi RP (2002) The alliance. In: Norcross JC (ed) Psychotherapy relationships that work: therapist contributions and responsiveness to patients. Oxford University Press, pp 37–69

Irwin A, Li J, Craig W, Hollenstein T (2016 Online, 2019 print) the role of shame in the relation between peer victimization and mental health outcomes. *Journal of Interpersonal Violence* 34(1): 156–181.

Kazantzis DN, Tee JM, Dattilio FM, Dobson KS (2017) The therapeutic relationship in cognitive behavior therapy: a clinician's guide. Guildford Press.

Lavender A (2019) Part 1, the therapeutic relationship in CBT. In: The therapeutic relationship in cognitive behavioural therapy. Sage, London.

Leary MR (1983) A brief version of the fear of negative evaluation scale. *Personality and Social Psychology Bulletin* 9:371–375

Lewis M (2003) The role of the self in shame. *Social Research* 70(4, Winter):1181–1204.

Mentalisation-based treatment: Basic training. (n.d.) Anna Freud Centre for Children and Families. http://www.annafreud.org/training-research/training-and-conferences-overview/training-at-the-anna-freud-national-centre-for-children-and-families/mentalisation-based-treatment-basic-training/

Prochaska JO, DiClemente CC, Norcross JC (1992) In search of how people change: applications to the addictive behaviours. *American Psychologist* 47:1102–1114

Rolland JS (2018) Helping couples and families navigate illness and disability: an integrated approach. Guildford Press, London, New York.

Scheier ME, Carver CS (1987) Dispositional optimism and physical well-being: the influence of generalized outcome expectancies on health. *Journal of Personality and Social Psychology* 55(2):169–210

Tomkins S (1963) Affect imagery consciousness. Vol II. The negative affects. Springer, New York.

Viladaga R, Hayes SC, Schelin L (2007) Philosophical, theoretical and empirical foundations of acceptance and commitment therapy. Anuario de Psicologica 38:117–128.

Vilardaga R, Hayes SC (2009) The therapeutic relationship stance. European Psychotherapy 9(1): 117–139.

7

Healing Conversations

Aspects of Self

This chapter focuses on establishing the therapeutic relationship and the process of accepting deficits and celebrating strengths. It will also consider the use of time in the context of therapeutic work.

There are not many therapists who haven't discovered, at some point in their agreed therapy plan, that they have started from the 'wrong' or less significant problem, or that somehow a key piece of information has not been mentioned. There is a whole literature on 'doorknob moments', and whatever else they indicate, they surely mean that something important has been buried or neglected. In both cases somehow until then the patient (or therapist) has not thought of it or found a moment to bring it up. Therapy may have initially appeared to go well, but when both therapist and client sideline a significant concern it is time for reflection.

© The Author(s) 2020
V. Purcell, *Understanding Visible Differences*, Palgrave Texts in Counselling and
Psychotherapy, https://doi.org/10.1007/978-3-030-51655-0_7

Co-creating Exclusion Zones

In some therapeutic approaches less is written about the therapist's own life experiences and the impact these can have on the relationship, whether they are spoken of or left unsaid. The impact of a client's words and the subtle interaction of non-verbal communication permit or deny awareness and exploration. Much is also inevitably left out given the time pressure of therapy, when even supervision can feel a hurried experience with many cases to discuss. A normal session plan will be 12 hours spread over 3–4 months, or 20 if it is a more complex case. Research shows that improvements are often gained in the first 4 sessions if the therapeutic alliance has been established, though time is needed for deeper and more resilient changes. This inevitably means that a lot of relevant and potentially useful information is not covered and could not be in the time available.

> As part of the assessment and planning it is worth talking about this. The question, 'do you think there is anything important/relevant we have not discussed?' should always be asked before formulation.
> Is it worth going further and saying something like—'Is there anything important that we might both avoid talking about, although it matters?' What could we do to avoid that?

Tools for Reflection

Time and Timelines

The use of Time as a therapeutic tool can be very powerful, whether working towards the therapy plan, processing challenging experiences, conversations or information, or reflecting on what has happened in the past using a timeline. Future and perspective-taking questions and those about the past concerning the impact of choice or events on the life path can reveal unresolved regrets and/or rumination.

The timeline is a very helpful tool for putting experiences into perspective and identifying patterns. Done together in session as part of the assessment it creates a form of visual narrative, capturing periods of time, organising events which may have been experienced as chaotic, or overwhelming. Like the genogram in systemic work, viewing it together affords an easier step towards discussing different perspectives, how things are, how they might change and how the client would like them to be different.

Adapting What Is Most Familiar, Rather Than Standard Formats

When considering approaches to the work find out what tools are most simple and familiar for your client—one idea might be to ask them how they have reflected on their self and their process in the past. Responses to this question are likely to be highly varied, with some only doing it when things go wrong, some keeping a regular journal. For many in the digital age social media or blogs may be part of this, and your client may agree to share some content which is helpful to the work, allowing a richer understanding of other aspects of self. People of strong faith might include self-reflection as part of their prayer and meditation to some extent, or this might be their only reference point to the question. Try asking yourself this question first! Are there particular moments or methods you prefer? How might you work with a person whose culture and beliefs focus strongly on duty and family honour rather than self?

> Decide with your client how they will record the work you do, and how you can contribute. For instance if you give handouts or links, how will they be included?

What Does Your Client Mean by 'Self'?

It is helpful to create an opportunity to talk about 'self' or different aspects of self as process rather than as a fixed object or set of characteristics, something they may or may not have thought about before. If they have been very organised towards external appearances and the expectations of others, this could be a novel experience. In considering how to do this, you of course need to consider the basic stability of the person's identity. Difficulties in the person's relationship with themselves are characteristic of mental health problems. In a therapy context you may be focusing on how a negative, uncertain or undermining pattern is being maintained. This may originally have been internalised from an external discourse, and be something 'uncovered' through diary work or something similar. This opens an opportunity to talk about how reflection tools can be elaborated in ways they will continue to find valuable. If they take up this suggestion and continue post-treatment, your clients have a better chance of remembering and continuing to use methods you have worked on in the therapy context, and more securely establishing changes they have made.

Central to this is the language used in relation to the self. Most of us are familiar with patterns of negative self-talk. In many cases they reference ideas about things in wider society, some of which they won't even agree with but have never focused on consciously. Typical of this is the belief 'I am worthless'. When time is taken in session to explore who else they think is worthless it is common to find that they don't really support the idea that anyone is worthless. They have simply put their attitude to themselves in a different box. More challenging can be clients who live in a social or cultural context where these beliefs are reinforced.

Don't forget the power of a visual metaphor—pictures and diagrams can reveal unexpected associations.

Maintain the Interest

Diary keeping and online communications can be utilised from the start of clinical work to begin to explore how often this happens, and clients can really feel liberated and energised by realising how often these subtle (or not-so-subtle) values pass un-noticed in the daily rain of media communications. Developing skills in challenging and defending against them, while building a positive dialogue with themselves is a gold standard life skill for all of us.

Differences in Power

The issue of power in the therapeutic relationship is rarely considered in training courses, with the exception of systemic approaches, and an inexperienced therapist using a more technological approach may not be in the habit of routinely considering how this is being constructed and reinforced in the clinical setting and therapy session. If a clinical training did not include a requirement for personal therapy, there may not be a lived understanding of what it is like to be in the client role. If you recognise this as a possible gap in your experience, consider making some time to reflect beyond your normal empathic pattern.

As a qualified therapist, whether working within an institution or independent professional your words carry authority, including the power to locate and define the problem. This is useful! But it should always be utilised in a considered way with an understanding of how your client receives it. It is often educational to ask your client to summarise the session before finishing, or perhaps take the lead in session later in the treatment plan.

If they find this difficult, it may be that they have become too passive in the therapy, and the 'relationship' so important to recovery has become one-sided.

Take Time for Reflection: What Is Really Going On?

The pressure recently qualified therapists feel to be excellent by sticking rigidly to the treatment manual also means that more 'doorknob' moments occur in the earlier part of a therapist's career, though they are always a possibility. This is one of the values of supervision, giving time to reflect on what is happening in an unspoken (or spoken) way. Even outside of supervision, listening to a recording of a session can yield a great deal of subtle information about the relationship that was missed at the time because the focus was on something else. For instance, I have listened to many recordings of therapy sessions where the therapist has asked the client about what they would like to talk about as part of agenda setting, the client has named an issue, and treatment is then focused else-where for the whole session! Of course, if your client brings a different crisis every week, you need to agree what is relevant to the work in order that the agreed work is not derailed. In addition, differences in age, gen-der and culture also create potential restrictions and misunderstandings which need to be processed somehow. Busy practices can leave little time for reflection, but this important time needs to be respected.

How might you create this in your working life?

For Therapeutic Gains to Last, They Must be Integrated Into Your Client's World of Meaning

Though the impact of truly 'meeting' your client in therapy can be tre-mendous, in the end what is discovered must continue to be relevant and accessible to them. In a multicultural context the issue described by Per Jensen (2016) as 'therapeutic colonisation' needs to be held in mind. Jensen draws on Habermas' (1987) concept of 'colonisation of the life world', referring to 'the background environment of competences, prac-tices and attitudes representable in terms of one's cognitive horizon'. This brings us to a complex ethical space, where the values and rights of the client and those whose lives they impact need to be carefully weighed. Again, careful reflection outside of the session is needed, especially as management of any potential issues should be as lightly done as possible, not laboured.

Is this something which can be added to your client's therapy diary in a routine way, or as part of review and ending?

Consider 'Staging' the Work If You Think Important Issues Might Arise Later

In developing a therapy plan with someone who has a visible difference the therapist should always make time to reflect on the possible impact looking different has/may have had on the presenting problem in a positive or negative way. This should be done in private, after the first assessment session, unless the patient brings it up. If the difference is congenital the client themselves may not always be fully aware of the interaction between their difference and the presenting issue. If you think this might be the case suggesting a 'review' session relatively early on can offer the opportunity for making connections when the therapeutic relationship is established. Your client may have found in the past that others avoid some of their questions because they are worried about hurting their feelings, or tell 'white lies' for the same reason, leaving them with doubts they can't voice. The therapy context can be a precious opportunity in this case. Similarly, when reviewing towards the end of therapy work the suggestion that issues can be revisited at a later life stage (if needed) is useful. Their diary work can be an invaluable resource.

What Has Been Avoided Can Be Brought Into the Conversation Using Third Party Material

The examples offered in this book, and references from film, books and media can be utilised to initiate a subject, or help you learn more about your client's perspective on things.

As part of the assessment process, consider what life stage they are in, their support systems, points of reference and any obvious unhelpful defences or sensitivities. What are their goals? Are they aiming low because they do not want to expose themselves to prejudice? Some people with visible differences can be very skilled at reading others, alert to possible threats and careful not to activate them. This avoidance can unnecessarily limit their lives without their being fully aware of it. It could also limit exchanges in the therapeutic context if they read the therapist as someone with unexamined attitudes. They are more likely to be comfortably honest about this with someone else who is different, so it is up to the therapist to create a space to discuss difference. Otherwise this can become 'the elephant in the room' with someone who has not fully considered connections with the issue, practices 'helpful' denial, or is habituated to issues. If you think this is extreme, or just illustrates the client's poor adjustment, consider whether you would make similar assumptions in their shoes if it was potential racial prejudice.

Some people now spend a lot of time in private working on their 'social media image'. You could suggest making this private rehearsal space a place for experimentation related to your therapeutic work (without posting the results). How might this work?

Celebrating Strengths and Resources

The first conversation about visible difference the therapist has with the client may be about how well they have met serious challenges so far, and an exploration of what helped them. How do they think of themselves in relation to others? Is self-esteem an issue in some circumstances? Do they privately find their friends or peers vain, thoughtless, or lacking in understanding at times? Taking the time to learn how they speak about experiences, and their relationship with themselves, in a sensitive and reflective exchange is the bedrock on which you can establish a shared language and understanding. This will give them the confidence to speak honestly about their concerns and take risks with change. The therapist will then find it much easier to move on to talk about things that have gone less well. This may seem obvious, but it can be much harder to recover the therapeutic relationship from an early setback. Some writers in this field have noted that clients who have not yet developed a positive coping response to staring and other forms of public humiliation tend to display anger rather than assertive responses (Clarke et al. 2014). While this clearly needs work, the therapist should bear in mind the link between internal shame and aggressive defence. Anger can be reframed as an attempt to assert the injustice of a situation, and the value of self. It is from this position that new approaches can be learned which help the person to remain balanced in situations where they had previously felt threatened. In this case early conversations need to be carefully managed, with good examples at hand. The (later) development of a compassionate stance towards the perpetrators, the coping strategies, and humour are eventual goals for a 'best life'.

Once again, role play, in session or privately, can be very helpful. Recordings are also a great opportunity to take a third party perspective.

Try to Be Honest with Yourself

In the current parlance of identity politics, it is also sometimes important for a therapist to 'check their privilege', noting privately any misplaced guilt, pity, patronising feelings and their own unresolved issues. For instance, are they someone who is very concerned with appearance, in real life and online, though they are in the 'normal' range? On first meeting did they feel some aversion to their client's appearance? Could they share this with their supervisor in order to understand and make it useful to the work? If not, they may need to reflect on whether this is likely to impact on their ability to help, and how it will be seen by the patient, who may habitually make comparisons which trigger self-criticism. Race, ethnicity, make up, hair colour and texture, clothing, visible disfigurement, body shape and size, all are relevant to working with body image concerns, and may need to be discussed. Difference of experience should not be a disqualification, but a consideration, opening the door for mutual growth. This may feel slightly controversial in an environment which is necessarily and rightly focused on the recovery of the client at all times. But most therapists acknowledge that they have learned a lot from their clinical interactions, and this is one of the rewards of the profession.

Apologise If You Get It Wrong

Comments which highlight the gulf in experience without offering empathic understanding may also trigger emotions of shame, anxiety or anger (sometimes interpreted as envy). Needless to say, this will disrupt the therapist's attempt to build an alliance and do a good assessment. The shame coping strategy of physical and psychological withdrawal was found to be the primary risk factor for developing a less effective alliance by Black et al. (2013). While these difficult emotions are very much part of later exploration to establish a different understanding of self, which may also include a compassion focus, at this stage they may cause disengagement without explanation.

For therapists unsure about the felt experience of visible difference, or seeking a way to discuss this with clients, literary resources can be very helpful, for instance Ishiguro's evocation of unacknowledged difference in 'Never Let Me Go', and sibling guilt in Hosseini's 'The Kite Runner'. Your client may well have books which have particularly resonated with their experiences, so this is worth asking about. Links with personal or religious philosophy can also be explored and evaluated for their helpfulness and accuracy as part of the change process, which may include schema work.

Reciprocal Resonance

This describes clinical conversations where the therapist's life experience and the client's share similar life events, optimally resulting in a therapeutic process where the relationship between the therapist and their client has the character of mutual understanding. Whether these are overtly discussed or not the sense of understanding and being understood will be present. However, if these overlaps have not been sufficiently processed by the therapist and the material being discussed is traumatic or aversive it can result in a personal crisis, instead of more positively a chance for the therapist to also share in learning from the dialogue. In this context the quality of the supervision relationship is very important (Jones 2003). Their supervisor can also help them consider whether they have fully reflected on their own projection of meaning and values into the therapeutic space, and whether the client is free from undue influence.

Whose Issue Are You Working On?

Few therapists would disagree with the idea that they have learned from their clients, though this is a situation not much discussed, but there is a professional responsibility on the therapist to ensure that they are not acting outside of their capacity to provide a safe environment for their client.

Research on the life experiences of American psychologists indicates that 30% of male and 70% of female psychologists report incidents of molestation or abuse in early life (in Harte Bratt 2019). 'Over identification, regression, personal resonance with what they hear compromising judgement, a tendency to be the rescuer or parent-surrogate, anxiety, depression and hopelessness are just a few on the long list of negative impacts clinical work may have on the therapist whose self-care is neglected.' The therapist needs to be able to recognise when their 'professional self' has been overwhelmed and take action. This may be in the form of managing the pace of the work, as the client may well be struggling too. In addition, an experienced supervisor and/or therapist can help to contain and process the work and even help them consider whether to continue.

What resources can you call upon if you find yourself in a similar situation?

Trauma

For a number of reasons, it is very important for clients to feel confident that the therapist has the ability to tolerate hearing their story, without being overwhelmed. It may be that they need reassurance on this point— telling them you have experience of listening to many difficult stories, though each one is unique, you have good supervisory support and so on. Your client may have had experiences of attempting to share with others when it has not gone well, and a stance of compassion and interest in what this was like for them is a good way to establish a safe base. As previously discussed, at the assessment stage (or later) unresolved trauma in relation to certain incidents may be disclosed, or more generalised distress which needs to be explored in a therapy setting and understood more helpfully. Telling the story, alongside a timeline for instance, can be a powerful intervention, but an assessment for PTSD symptoms should also be made and the treatment plan adjusted accordingly. In some cases, it may be necessary to postpone the first treatment plan and focus on PTSD work first.

Sometimes narrative work encompassing multiple trauma events can be more successful (Schauer et al. 2011). As in any trauma work the story needs to be told by beginning from a safe point and ending at a safe point. This is the case even if the narrative needs to be returned to in order to further explore particularly painful incidents as well as to work on the trauma. Also, the clients processing of the therapy experience between sessions (and any reflections that arise) should be a starting point next time. This helps the client to feel in control, and to manage their fears of being overwhelmed by what they are saying. (Grey 2013)

Although the concept of post-traumatic growth (Calhoun et al. 2010) has been called into question by some recent research, there is no doubt that over time individuals can respond to very challenging events by developing wisdom, understanding, strength and compassion. This does take time though, and an alternative explanation is that people may quickly feel as if they are better people without being so, as a defensive response. Experimental studies, which focus on relatively recent trauma in student populations, have found that belief in post-traumatic growth can reflect a coping strategy to minimise and manage distress and not actual change.

Most of us are familiar with the Nietzsche quote 'that which does not kill us, makes us stronger'. A strengths and resilience approach should not deny the reality of losses, rather foster the recognition that there is scope for the development of a different perspective and depth of character in adversity. As noted in previous chapters, children often respond to being different by longing to be normal. It takes further, more complex, cognitive and personal development to see value (and humour) in their different status. A more mature stance might be the acceptance of both perspectives.

Supportive Reciprocal Resonance

Supportive reciprocal resonance (Dallos and Vetere 2009) can be regarded as a secure base for therapy providing the opportunity for the client to take a new direction, learning in the relationship. It describes the elements of the therapists' personal and private lives which are utilised in the therapy context during their interaction with clients, and which resonate with their clients understanding and experiences in a way which facilitates helpful change.

Indeed, of the multitude of factors that account for success in psychotherapy, clinicians of different orientations converge on this point: the therapeutic relationship is the cornerstone. (Norcross 2010)

Self-compassion and the development of healthy self-love are the active goals of this process. Earlier therapeutic work on resilience and coping skills can facilitate movement between aspects of self (the immersed person-in-the-moment telling their story and the mature caring adult self hearing it) that leads to greater resolution and stability.

The purpose is to establish a relationship in which the meaning of 'normal' can be redefined without denial, shame triggers can be identified, the shame-givers power to define undermined, and strategies for managing the challenges of difference can be strengthened or established in relation to the presenting problems. Then the client's life can be lived as fully as possible. As previously noted, a secure identity less focused on external appearances, plus strategies and ways of living which develop and maintain resilience are needed for positive mental health. Part of this work may be helping them engage more with other online voices and/or real-time sources of social support, online therapy and recovery accounts, for example that of Katie Piper, whose recovery has been very much enacted in the media (see Katie Piper Foundation). These resources can enhance what the therapist is able to offer and create a supportive bridge after treatment.

> Once again, a timeline is your ally in constructing the understanding that this development will continue. Your client can place themselves on this continuum, and you can reflect together on what future life experiences will draw them on.

Reciprocal Resilience

This refers to the capacity of the therapist, client and their therapeutic relationship to manage the therapeutic tasks in front of them. Resilience is defined as 'the ability of a substance to return to its usual shape after being bent, stretched or pressed' or with reference to humans 'the ability to be happy, successful etc. again after something difficult or bad has happened' (Cambridge Dictionary). Both definitions refer to a return to previous form, though I would argue that therapy's better moments allow for something more transformative, and this is what this book aims to address. This is the reach forward to different and maybe greater possibilities, where things that have been avoided, discounted or given up can be worked towards and achieved. This could be a bit grand, and it is true that accepting objective circumstances is an important part of therapeutic work. But in this acceptance, other things can become possible. If you no longer worry about what you look like on the dance floor you are free to let rip and fully enjoy it. Or at least dance in the dark and feel free.

Good Days and Bad Days

For both therapist and client there are good days and bad days. While this could be a chapter of its own, reflecting on our own management of low confidence and low energy days, and being honest about it with clients (where helpful and relevant) can really help in the development of sustainable long-term strategies for living with visible difference.

Central to recovery is the task of building resilience, firstly noting skills and capacities that are well developed, and then identifying situations which are more difficult. What is it about those situations which make accessing personal resources more difficult? Challenging beliefs and modifying behaviours means using existing capacities to build new skills and strengths. But even a strong and confident sense of self can be really challenged by prejudiced others, and it is important to both frankly acknowledge that they exist and have a variety of outline plans for how to deal with them. Including walking away sometimes without feeling bad about yourself, and occasionally being selective in friendships. Biases may be at a social or cultural level and give rise to the question of who should own the 'problem' of difference. In all cases allowing shame and anxiety to limit the full development of the self is one cause of unhappiness. Recovery comes from a realistic appraisal of the challenges (internal and external) and the development of resources to cope without unnecessary restriction. We are fortunate to live in a time and place where change is happening around us. There are great examples in the media and many more ways to connect with like-minded others who can share their informed support.

References

Black SA, Curran D, Dyer KFW (2013) The impact of shame on the therapeutic alliance and intimate relationships. Wiley Online Library. https://doi.org/10.1002/jclp.21959

Calhoun LG, Cann A, Tedeschi RG (2010) The post-traumatic growth model: sociocultural considerations. In: Weiss T, Berger R (eds) Post-traumatic growth and culturally competent practice: Lessons learned from around the globe. John Wiley and Sons Inc., Hoboken, NJ, pp 1–14

Clarke A, Thompson AR, Jenkinson E, Rumsey N, Newell R (2014) CBT for appearance anxiety: psychosocial interventions for anxiety due to visible difference. Wiley Blackwell

Dallos R, Vetere A (2009) Systemic therapy and attachment narratives: applications in a range of settings. Routledge, London

Grey N (ed) (2013) A casebook of cognitive therapy for traumatic stress reactions. Routledge

Harte Bratt P (2019) Mutual growth in the psychotherapeutic relationship: reciprocal resilience. Routledge

Jensen P (2016) Mind the map. In: Vetere A, Stratton P (eds) Interacting selves: systemic solutions for personal and professional development in counselling and psychotherapy. Routledge

Jones E (2003) Working with the 'self' of the therapist in consultation. *Human Systems* 14(1):7–16

Norcross JC (2010) The therapeutic relationship. In: Duncan BL, Miller SD, Wampold BE, Hubble MA (eds) The heart and soul of change: delivering what works in therapy, 2nd edn. American Psychological Association, Washington, DC, pp 113–141

Schauer M, Neuner F, Elbert T (2011) Narrative exposure therapy: a short-term treatment for traumatic stress disorders. Hogrefe

8

Thinking About Treatment Plans and Models: A Formulation-Based Approach

Developing the formulation together is a powerful intervention, building understanding, containment and hope in the client, plus a greater interest in and respect for themselves. It can be used as a starting point for change, though alongside this there must be awareness of the possible need to recognise and grieve the lost or injured self, whether this is real or imagined. This may be the first stage of the work.

Assessment of the client's current resilience strategies (when they work well, and when they fail) is part of considering changes that they would like to achieve. As is the possibility of post-traumatic growth, achieved and anticipated, as one of the helpful by-products of working through and coming to terms with difficult experiences, though consider if this is being used as a defence. How will they be different at the end of this process? Many of the people I have met and interviewed who are different are proud of their achievements in living life against the grain of beauty bias, though it can also be wearing and there are good and bad days.

The process of formulation will of course take different forms, depending on the therapeutic approach, and it is not the aim of this book to direct the reader to one. Rather, to invite consideration of different approaches likely to be useful and tools which might be used coherently

© The Author(s) 2020
V. Purcell, *Understanding Visible Differences*, Palgrave Texts in Counselling and Psychotherapy, https://doi.org/10.1007/978-3-030-51655-0_8

within a treatment plan, to improve the outcome. Each different model has a slightly different focus and strengths, depending on their interpretation of the problem and what is needed to help the client. In all cases though there are basic categories of information that will be important (Fig. 8.1).

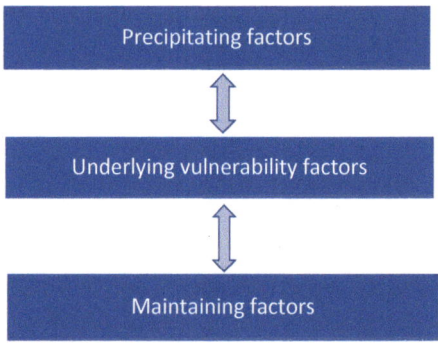

Fig. 8.1 Factors for treatment plans

Developing an Individual Formulation-Based Approach to Treatment

While many treatment approaches are based on an initial formulation, sometimes reformulated as therapy progresses, what is considered here is how you might tailor this approach to your client's unique presentation, while retaining a coherent and productive treatment plan.

All will begin with assessment measures, identification of the problem(s) to be worked on and agreed treatment goals. At the same time, a **systemic stance** beginning with developing a map of the client's interpersonal world and their relationships will help you to establish how their relationship with themselves, their thoughts and feelings fit and are shaped by their social context. This is particularly important when you have a client who experiences themselves and is seen by others as 'different'. It could be considered a form of continued distortion or abuse to locate the problem entirely within the individual, without mapping the context of their difficulties, and naming what should be situated outside of the person.

The initial time frame for the work is also agreed, and any planned breaks like holiday discussed alongside confidentiality and cancellation policies. You may also consider whether some sessions will be conducted online, also time spent reviewing logs and other information/messages from the client outside of the therapy session.

Getting the emphasis right—An accurate and careful individual formulation, which identifies the skills, resources and resilience the client has, as well as correctly identifying problems and goals can be referenced throughout the treatment. Getting the emphasis right is something that should be revisited as therapy progresses to ensure it is still fit for purpose. For instance, by starting with a problem list and an active approach to setting useful tasks between sessions right from the first, one can help to establish a commitment to the work. What counts as a 'task' depends on what is being done, it might be to find out a new piece of information about a person's early life to improve understanding, an imaginal exercise, or any other helpful thing you both agree on. Questions which facilitate different types of perspective taking can begin to stimulate curiosity—what might other people think if they said/did/changed/ in this or that way?

Doing what works and is compatible with your client's way of thinking and being—As previously stated more than one treatment approach can be effective, when within our competencies. As therapists we are all attracted by the promise of better, more effective treatment for our clients, and rightly so. When things get stuck we may anxiously wonder whether the choices made were optimal, and large data samples can offer good guidance on what works. The evidence-based approach to change is one of humanity's better ideas, hard to disagree with, a bit like 'an end to poverty'. Who will stand against it? Randomised Controlled Trials are the gold standard for research and where conducted provide good guidance. But they are also very expensive, so not enough are done to test all possible alternatives.

Research on what good therapists actually do in therapy demonstrates that they have many similarities, being skilled in focusing on what works for their patient, and often adapt their working models accordingly. It is also important to remember that RCTs can only provide statistical data on what works best from the few protocols that have been tested, in controlled conditions, often based on single issue presentations which are selected very carefully, and most real—life presentations are usually more complex. This is not an invitation to ignore research, though your own outcome data, in frank discussion with your supervisor will be most informative.

Where there is reason to doubt the effectiveness of your treatment plan, I would argue that the best evidence is gathered from your client. This requires a strong and honest therapeutic relationship, so that you can speak about the meaning of avoidance, procrastination, and so on. Of course, fidelity to tried and tested models is the primary option, but if it is not working for your individual client reflect on this and try to understand why.

Since the adoption of CBT in NICE (National Institute for Health and Care Excellence) guidelines many therapists trained in other models have acquired CBT skills but may feel less confident in integrating them in a treatment plan. Most research trials have focused on CBT and schema approaches, with less reliable outcome data on emerging third wave CBT therapies like Compassion Focused therapy and Acceptance and Commitment therapy. These seek to integrate approaches like compassion and mindfulness to improve the client's relationship with themselves and tolerance of emotion while retaining a focus on change. Categories of therapies tend to evolve, absorbing other pre-existing approaches which are recognised as useful, inevitably often in advance of supporting research studies—currently the wide application of the mindfulness approach is an example of this.

Styles of Formulation

It hardly needs to be said that the formulation style will be shaped by the underlying theory and focus of the treatment model, and where there is a choice, the client's preference and capacities.

For example, in Interpersonal Therapy for depression (offered by the NHS) the formulation is a spoken or written summary of what the client has told the therapist during assessment, constructed in a way which facilitates treatment. In Cognitive Analytic Therapy it is a diagram, created through the treatment period, which seeks to identify both the conscious and out of awareness processes impacting the client. Formulation in systemic therapies is always tentative and emerging, as such they are less proscriptive, focusing on how systems develop helpful and unhelpful patterns of interaction and meaning. Below we return to the formulation style in three of the models already discussed in relation to the therapeutic relationship.

A CBT formulation is frequently summarised within diagrams, tailored to a specific presenting problem which has a treatment protocol. This has the effect (ideally) of capturing and clarifying the patient's experience of the difficulties and creating the possibility of a pathway to change. The basic formulation is used to understand specific trigger situations and what maintains patterns of thoughts, feelings and behaviour, so that this cycle can be modified. A simple example follows (Fig. 8.2).

Techniques for modification include an exploration of maintaining beliefs in relation to the problem, challenging these where they are problematic, through evidence gathering often in behavioural experiments, and modification of underlying schemas through reformulation. There are a variety of techniques used to support this basic approach, for instance socratic dialogue, eliciting negative automatic thoughts, identifying and manipulating safety behaviours, and cost-benefit

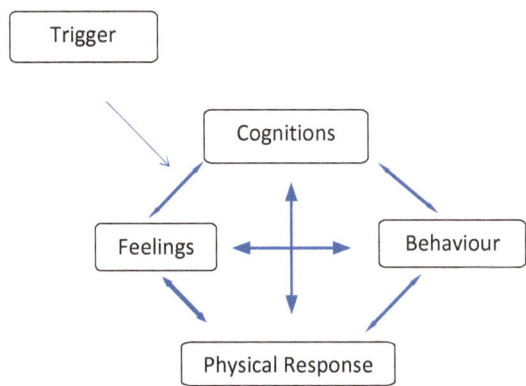

Fig. 8.2 CBT basic formulation example

analysis. Functional analysis may also be used to explore how and why a client has developed a pattern of beliefs and behaviours, with a view to modifying it.

Formulating in Compassion Focused Therapy—This approach was first developed in the early twenty-first century by Paul Gilbert (2010) and colleagues to help those suffering from high levels of self-criticism and shame. It is an integrative approach which uses tools from evolutionary theory, neuroscience and Buddhism, as well as psychology. The basic formulation used is slightly different from CBT, and looks at the threat response to identified problems (fight, flight and freeze) and related emotions, and how that interacts with other aspects of the self, imagery and visualization. It identifies three key affect systems.

The threat system is protection focused. It scans for threats and it's linked with anxiety, anger and the fight/flight response.

The drive system is excitement focused and motivates people to attain rewards and resources. It is associated with arousal, stimulation and achievement.

The contentment system is focused on soothing. It is triggered when there is no threat and we feel safe and socially connected. Feelings associated with this system are ones of calmness, contentment and peace.

A compassion-focused formulation will focus on these three areas and explore how they are interacting in relation to the problem and the client's relationship with themselves. Formulation will be in a series of steps, beginning with current problems and symptoms, making sense of these difficulties, and establishing the therapeutic relationship. As part of this, areas of difficulty are noted. This will be followed later in the work by a series of developments to the formulation, as the work progresses. The strength of this formulation is that (with help) many clients are readily able to recognise when their threat system is activated, and how that influences beliefs and behaviour (Fig. 8.3).

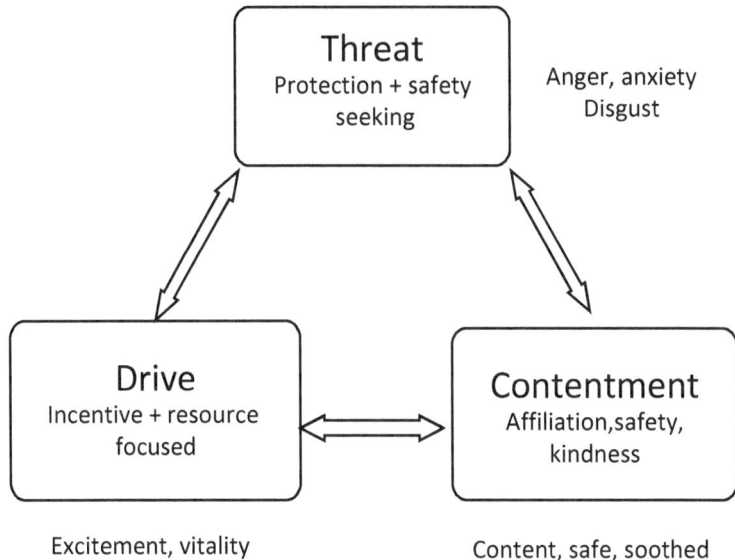

Fig. 8.3 Three areas formulation diagram

Formulation in Acceptance and Commitment therapy—ACT is a values-based behaviour therapy which uses acceptance and mindfulness interventions alongside commitment and behaviour change strategies. It aims to increase the client's ability to choose different approaches to problems through mindfully accepting their thoughts and feelings as they are rather than attempting to change them which often causes 'stuck' responses and prevents taking the risk of change. The development of acceptance and diffusion skills encourage contact with psychological content which is difficult and helps to create a sense of self which is distinct from and not threatened by challenging content. The model seeks to help the client understand what works for them, to accept what is happening and be more flexible. It is particularly helpful to clients who have been stuck in avoidant patterns that prevent them from doing things they in fact value highly.

A key technique is to work with the client to identify the values which are most important to them, and they wish to be identified with. This may use the 'miracle question' 'if you woke up tomorrow and discover you have achieved everything that matters to you in life. You feel 100% confident and happy. What would others see about you that is different Metcalf (2004)?'

There are many variations on this question and it is used in many models. A related technique to uncover values is to work with a values list and ask clients to select those that reflect how they would like to be thought of or remembered by others. These core values then serve to help the client focus on ways they wish to change or develop themselves through committed action, which may initially involve tolerating levels of discomfort previously avoided.

The key aspects are simply described by Sinclair and Beadman (2016) as 'wake up' (cultivate awareness), 'loosen up' (respond to thoughts and feelings in a looser, more accepting way) and 'step up' (stay focused on values-based meaning and fulfilment) when making changes in order to achieve more flexibility in relation to life circumstances while remaining focused on values which are important.

All these approaches offer ways to understand 'the problem(s)' and pathways to change. Resources are easily available online. Learningact.com has therapist materials for ACT, as does compassionatemind.co.uk, and getselfhelp.co.uk for CBT, acat.me.uk for CAT.

Co-create the Formulation

The exact nature of the formulation created will of course depend on the therapist's training and skill set. A more inclusive approach can be developed at the start, which focuses on the most salient issue, while understanding the connections to other related problems, and the patterns of thought, feeling and behaviour which link them. Whatever the form that the formulation takes it should be a summary which is experienced as clarifying and powerful for the client. Often this is one of the most significant interventions, which therapist and patient will return to during the treatment process (sometimes when they feel overcome by complexity). It is most helpful to write it down and keep the document available, and it should include in a balanced way the resources, resilience and skills the client brings to the task at that moment, as well as identifying those that need to be developed. The client should have a copy, and it is very important to process what it is like for the client to see it written in that way. Their reaction will often tell you whether you have got it right.

A question might help as both of you discuss the formulation you have created—you could for instance say, 'looking at this, can you think of anything important that we have not included, which might make a difference to our plan?'

Encourage your client to take some time to reflect on this. Therapists often experience that clients minimise abuse at assessment, in fact they may not mention it at all if it is out of immediate awareness. It is not until supervisor and therapist are wondering together why treatment is not working as they hoped it would that the possibility of underlying trauma is considered.

Putting This Into Practice: Three Examples

Authors note—case examples used have been anonymised and are not based on single cases to protect patient confidentiality.

Case Study 1: A Compassion and Shame Focus

Sarah, aged 23 has burns scarring, resulting from a kitchen accident when she was 5 years old. She has burns on the right arm and lower right side of her body. These can mostly be covered by clothing, and she makes sure that no-one except her closest friends ever sees the extent of them. She and her family had support during her recovery, but she does not remember much about it now. While she was always self-conscious about showing her scars around people she did not know, this became more pronounced in her early teens. She decided to focus on close friendships and study, doing well and getting into university, followed by entry straight into a graduate scheme. Sarah came to therapy to improve her close relationship confidence, as she has not dated anyone, avoiding all potentially romantic situations. She has so far explained this to others as a need to focus on developing her career, and friends and family joke about her independence and 'high standards'. She privately thinks she could not cope with rejection. Her parents divorced when she was young, and her mother remarried when she was 9. She is the only child of the first relationship and rarely sees her father who has also remarried, though he financially supported her studies. She describes her stepfather as 'OK'.

Sarah has one younger half- sister who is very outgoing, now at university and two older stepbrothers (+3 and +5) who are independent. They teased her about her burns, calling her a reptile when younger. She sees them infrequently but is in regular contact with her mother and aunts.

She is aware that she carefully controls all social interactions and feels quite envious of friends who she sees as more relaxed and 'free', especially their travel photos with bikinis and shorts, seen on social media. She has tried and enjoyed skiing and surfing as they both offer full cover outfits. In a professional situation she is confident and manages some 'banter' but avoids all situations where she might feel 'exposed', preferring to set the agenda. Her treatment goals are to be more socially confident and adventurous, go to a summer festival with friends, and agree to a date if someone she really likes invites her. When considering readiness, she stated that she was 'good to go!'

Her assessment scores showed she was moderately depressed and anxious.

Sarah's Problem List

1. Worry that she was not physically loveable—low self-esteem in this area.
2. Controlling situations to avoid risk.
3. Pressuring herself to compete, self-criticism, little 'downtime'.
4. Distancing herself from others.
5. Missing out on relationship chances, loneliness.
6. Later she added drinking on her own at home on the weekends.

Sarah's Strengths

She is motivated, wants to live her 'best life' and can see that to do this she needs to accept herself as she is.

Capable and ambitious, she has confidence in this work self.

Clear about what she wants.

Aware she is confident and likeable in some social situations.

Sarah's Social Map shows that she has a wide range of acquaintances, is active on social media, but has few close friends that might act as a 'wing man/woman'. The ones she did have are now in other parts of the country, so she does not see them much. In the past she has not identified with burns organisations, wanting to just get on with her life. Her mother is the person she is most likely to confide in.

The process of assessment seemed to go well, though the therapist felt quite 'managed', and she appeared uninterested in talking too much about the past. Having noted some self-critical attitudes, her therapist offered a suggestion that her thoughts, feelings and protective behaviours relating to her appearance might be maintaining an internal feeling of threat in some social situations, as part of a consideration of different ways to formulate this. Later they drew out the model below, while considering a compassion focused approach. When discussing it with Sarah, and how it felt to see it drawn out in that way, her initial response was lukewarm, saying she did not want to wallow in difficult feelings. This was not encouraging, but it led on to a discussion about what she felt was in the way of just doing the things she wanted, identifying the personal strengths and resources she had developed to support her.

Her answer was 'I am afraid of the exposure'.

Therapist: 'What do you imagine happening?'

Sarah: 'People I'm attracted to will look at my scars and feel sorry for me, or repulsed. I'm not sure which is worse, but I won't be able to cope.'

Therapist: 'That sounds like a pretty good reason for avoiding those situations! It sounds as if one of your fears about coming to therapy is that it might expose you to feelings you are not sure you can cope with.'

Previously Sarah had seen herself as 'good to go', so together they drew a simple timeline, looking at what would be the same or different if she continued with her current coping strategies, versus taking risks with change.

From this both were able to agree that an interim goal was to improve her confidence that she would be able to cope, and a discussion of options followed. The therapist offered the suggestion that if she wanted to extend her coping strategies, then maybe an initial focus on observing her thoughts and feelings without changing them might be helpful, as a baseline. But to begin with they agreed a few trials of trying to tell herself to 'cheer up', 'just relax' and 'don't get afraid' would be informative before the next meeting. They both wrote down predictions about what might happen, to compare next time with what did happen (Fig. 8.4).

At the next meeting, unsurprisingly Sarah had found her strategies to change her feelings had not worked, and she had noticed how tiring and frustrating it had been. She reported being aware of her feelings more

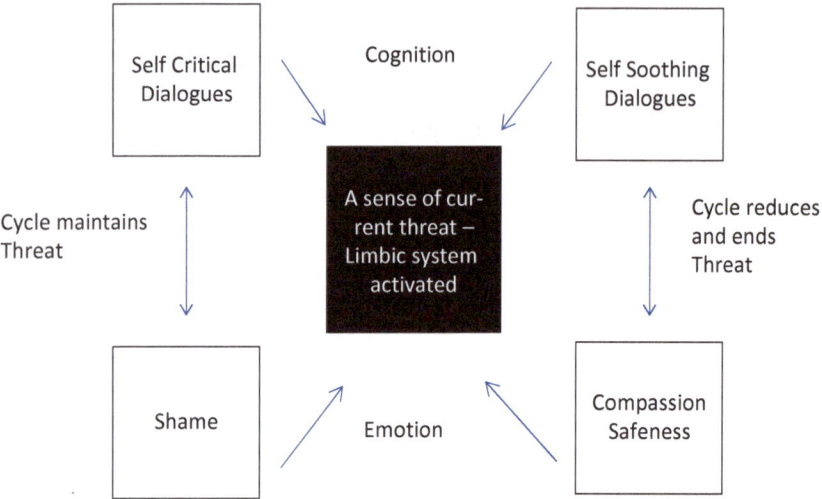

Fig. 8.4 Diagram adapted from Lee (2009)

which was uncomfortable but felt able to agree to try a mindfulness practice in session, to continue noticing and naming without trying to change her thoughts and feelings. She was not very keen to explore them in session. They agreed that she would continue to practice this before the next session and talked about whether she would be interested in seeking out some Facebook posts by burns survivors and if she felt like it a discussion forum.

Next session she reported that she had been surprised by what she found, having deliberately not looked before. In particular, the way people shared photos of their experiences and burns and supported each other. She talked about how that felt to her, saying she admired their courage and what it might feel like to the person posting those images and talking about it. Looking at the formulation again, she could see that the people concerned might be shifting away from a threat-based approach to coping, allowing themselves to receive different feedback, though she could not imagine doing that herself.

When discussing what would need to change Sarah found herself remembering her stepbrother's comments when they saw her burns, and she unexpectedly began to cry (saying 'I never do this!'). When it was possible to share this memory her therapist said 'looking back, what

Table 8.1 Her treatment diagram looked something like this

1	1	1								
2	2	2	2							
	3	3	3	3	3	3	3	3	3	3
				4	4	4	4	4	4	
							5	5	5	

Key—1 = Assessment and formulation; 2 = Introduction to the model and experiential work; 3 = Review of practice, analysis and restructuring; 4 = Schema and cognitive modification, exposure work; 5 = Relapse prevention and maintenance planning

might have helped you then, what did you need to know, or hear? They worked together on imagining an 'ideal helper', the conversation that might have taken place, and how that might have changed things. Sarah was very engaged by this, and able to recognise (with her therapist's help) that this compassionate and helpful voice was her own adult self. They agreed to continue with this imaginal practice between sessions.

Next session she was more understanding and less threatened by the compassion focused formulations, which formed the basis of the first part of treatment, with more emphasis on CBT based exposure work in the latter half (Table 8.1).

On her own initiative Sarah talked to her brother about some of her memories and difficulties next time she saw him, and (now much older and more caring) he was surprised and ashamed at the impact his behaviour had on her. This disclosure led to a better relationship, and she found that she enjoyed his company. Later he became her 'wing man' for some behavioural experiments.

For clients like Sarah the use of imagery can also be very helpful when the work moves towards a behaviour change focus, enabling them to 'rehearse' new experiences in a less threatening way, and then work with the therapist on strategies for areas where the visualization gets 'stuck'.

Case Study 2: ACT and CBT, Schema Work

James is 45 and recently divorced from his wife of 20 years, after she disclosed an affair and left. They had met and married when he was a young soldier and have two daughters who are now adults. He was later posted to Afghanistan, where he was seriously injured. He lost a leg and has facial scarring as well as some difficulties in using his right hand. Rehabilitation was a lengthy process and once discharged from the army he found it hard to get retraining and work. He now works in logistics, mainly from home. He was previously proud of his physical prowess, enjoying sports and outdoor activities, and later participated in some disabled sports though recently he has lost interest. Since the injury he has experienced periods of depression and low self-esteem and had very much relied on his wife to organise their social and family engagements. He is still devastated by her departure though she left 2 years ago. With the encouragement and support of his daughters he goes to the pub with a few ex-army friends occasionally and takes the dog out. All his daughter's efforts to get him to meet new people have been resisted and seem to have made him more gloomy. He says that they don't understand, and no-one is interested in an old bloke with one leg and scars.

They suggested he went to the GP as he is very anxious in social situations outside the family and has started drinking more heavily at home since the divorce was finalised, and he was referred for therapy. His elder daughter, who lives nearby, went with him to the GP, where she broke down in tears, upset at her parent's divorce and worried about him, which was the reason he accepted the referral. She also came with him to the first session.

The first therapist was a young woman. He appeared uncomfortable and uncommunicative throughout the assessment meeting, and after talking it through with his daughter and GP he requested a male therapist, emphasising it was not the first therapist's fault. After consideration he was offered another assessment with a man closer to his own age, which he said he found more helpful.

James' assessment scores showed depression in the severe range, and low self-esteem. He acknowledged suicidal ideation, and had thought of shooting himself, but said he was unlikely to act because his daughters still needed him. A safety contract was agreed.

His problem list
Depression, low motivation.
Loneliness.
Feels he has no future.

Believes he is boring.

His goals

Support his daughters and not worry them (this was all that he could identify).

When asked the 'miracle question' James first replied that his injuries would disappear.

His therapist then asked him to identify what difference that would make. He replied, 'I would feel more confident, more like a man, and I would probably still be married'. Following this they worked on exploring the differences between James before his injuries and afterwards, apart from physical changes.

> James has several interconnecting serious problems, and the therapist's first task is to ensure he remains safe and has sufficient support and resilience to cope with the challenges of therapy. He appears to be grieving both for his lost self and his marriage.
>
> His therapist asked him to keep a mood and activity log, and agreed to focus early session time mainly on grief work. The logs were used to identify times in the week when he felt better/worse, and any association with behaviours. In addition, the therapist continued to make notes on his patterns of thought, and links with behaviours.

He said he felt that although he has worked hard at rehabilitation, and his wife was very supportive, he did not really like himself after that, and it had affected their physical relationship. He wondered if she just felt sorry for him, and still does. He sometimes felt angry and resented his friends who came through the war unscathed (though he hid it). This made him feel like a bad person.

His therapist noted that when he talked about his life post injury, it seemed as if he felt he had failed, and wondered aloud about this. James agreed, but then in further discussion recognised he could not have avoided what happened without letting his comrades down. He agreed that this didn't make sense, though he couldn't see how he could feel differently. During this the therapist was noting his thoughts, feelings and behaviours on paper, so that they could be seen, later linking this with his activity and mood logs.

This simple beginning helped James to express and tolerate his difficult feelings and structure his days in a way that improved his mood and activity levels. Though the underlying patterns of thought had not changed he was able to disrupt them through changing behaviours, and not fall into a 'black hole' as he described it.

At this point the therapist returned to explore his relationship with himself, noting his tendency to negativity about his changed appearance, predictions about other's opinions of him, and defensive, avoidant patterns of behaviour. Beginning to formulate this, they identified some of his rules for living, which had not altered since before his injuries, a time when his self-esteem was based on his physical skills and competence, as well as his looks (being very attractive to women). His recovery from injury had focused on areas of competence and developing new skills, but his success seemed to have been based in part on relentlessly bullying himself (for perceived weakness) when he felt like giving up, a pattern now contributing to suicidal feelings. Using Fennell's (1997) cognitive model of low self-esteem as a framework to explore the earlier pattern, James could see how his divorce had confirmed his bottom line, activating depression, negative predictions, self-criticism and hopelessness, together with several unhelpful behaviours. It also made clear that the basis for this unhelpful pattern was there already, but to compensate he had used his appearance as a confidence booster, a strategy he felt was unavailable since then.

James reflected on how his wife and family had in some ways provided a solution for his social anxieties, a readymade social buffer, meaning that he could avoid making some adjustments. This seems harsh but was typical of James' judgements of himself. His therapist wondered with him whether a compassion focus was needed, but first using a functional analysis of his approach they looked at what had been helpful about that for him at the time, and how his previous method of motivating himself (self-criticism) had now become an overlooked problem that needed to be attended to. As he rarely acknowledged his resilience and coping skills his therapist took the opportunity to draw his attention to them, noting the ways they had been enhanced through his recovery and adjustment. Together they explored possible methods of healing his divided inner relationship, though James was initially uncomfortable with a compassion model saying it felt like 'making excuses for himself'. They agreed on a resilience focus and good/bad day structure, as a shame-attacking strategy, and created a combined formulation which included his social anxiety and low self-esteem. However, his therapist wanted to keep a focus on emotion, and suggested a short regular mindfulness practice, beginning in session.

The reader will have noticed that James' judgement of his appearance has not so far been a treatment focus, though it has not been ignored. At this point in the therapy there is a good therapeutic alliance, and his therapist has been carefully cataloguing aspects of James that were attractive and nothing to do with physical appearance. While earlier encouragement to be more socially active had kept James in his social comfort zone, it seemed the right moment to talk about whether he wanted to meet new people (Table 8.2).

His therapist used a timeline as a tool for this purpose, 0–100, locating his achievements, children, injury, marriage and divorce along it, and suggested that regardless of his injury this would be a moment of re-evaluation in his life. Addressing his belief that he was boring, they identified thoughts and behaviours that tended to reinforce it. The next step was some values work, clarifying what was important to him now and going forward, and how he wanted to be seen by others in different life

Table 8.2 His treatment diagram looked like this—(20+ sessions) TBA

1	1	1												
2	2	2	2											
		3	3	3	3	3	3	3	3	3	3	3	3	
				4	4	4	4	4	4	4	4	4	4	4
												5	5	5

Key—1 = Assessment and grief work; 2 = Introduction to the basic CBT model, logs and behavioural activation; 3 = Review and formulation, functional analysis and restructuring of self-concept; 4 = Schema and cognitive modification, exposure work; 5 = Relapse prevention and maintenance planning areas. This created new goals well beyond the completion of therapy. Addressing his own prejudice towards himself, and that he anticipated from others was part of this. James was ready to do it, though not put himself 'out there'.

Committing to his values and using his resilience and skills James decided to volunteer as a supporter for disabled sport. He found this very satisfying, particularly with younger people who he enjoyed being around and this new context allowed him to work on his social confidence. It also brought him into contact with their parents, some of whom were his age, which was mutually beneficial.

Though this was a complex journey, James had the skills, love and determination he needed to connect with and realise his important values, creating new goals for the second half of his life. He stopped thinking he was boring.

Case Study 3: CBT and Trauma

Anita is a young woman, aged 30 who was born with a facial port wine stain. It is lighter following laser treatment, but has not gone, and Anita has heard it may also worsen in later life, requiring more treatment. She was bullied as a child because of her appearance, both at home by her elder siblings, and at school, and she initially presents as composed but reserved. Her uncle sexually abused both her and a cousin, and it was her cousin who disclosed this first seven years ago. There has been a court case, in which she reluctantly gave evidence to support her cousin and the uncle went to prison. It was a huge shame for the family, and nobody talked about it now. Anita had some trauma-related therapy after that. She tells her therapist that when she was younger she just wanted to forget about it all, and leave it behind her. She left home as soon as she could and always uses concealing makeup. But she now wants therapy to 'resolve it all' so that she can have a lasting relationship without rushing to the bathroom in the morning to do her makeup. She would like to have a family later with someone who can accept her.

She lives independently and works as a microbiologist and is confident of her skills in this area, though she feels that she loses out sometimes in office politics. Apart from work contacts she is involved in a cycling group, and travels with arranged groups. She manages her social media presence, occasionally writes an anonymous blog about surviving abuse, is regularly involved in online gaming and has been since university. She also attends 'Comicon' events where she dresses as Alita Battleangel (a cyberpunk manga character) and has an online presence where she talks about developing the costume.

None of her current work or former uni friends know the abuse that happened to her, and she explains that at university (where she did see a counsellor for social anxiety) it didn't seem like something she could share. Later, the time was never right. Her counsellor did not mention her birthmark, (she thinks because she always wore makeup) and neither did she.

Anita has 2 previous episodes of treatment. The first she describes as 'counselling' following the abuse trial, and she says that it helped her to talk about what happened and realise that she was not to blame.

The second was CBT for social anxiety, and this helped her to speak up in seminars, and go out socially with her flatmates. She had a serious boyfriend at uni, but since then a 'couple of flings' and hook-ups.

A timeline was used as part of assessment, also noting resilience factors and coping strategies. Assessment scores show mild low mood, and anxiety, and there was no evidence of flashbacks, startle response or other obvious trauma symptoms.

Anita's problem list
Ending relationships if they might get more serious.
Lack of 'relationship skills' (her words).
Trust in intimate relationships.
Periods of crying and withdrawal.
Anxiety about others seeing her birthmark.
Her goals
Put the past behind me.
Feel more confident (including without makeup).
Stay in a relationship and have the skills to make it work.
Not be anxious and distrustful.

On meeting Anita she appeared to have coped well with the challenges in her life so far, though at some cost, as some aspects of her were carefully protected.

Anita's social map showed a close group of supportive friends who she had fun with. Her mother, cousin and one university friend were the people she was most likely to confide in. Later she described her mother as a worrier though and said she did not want to upset her by talking about problems too much. Her brother was now married, and her younger sister had a serious boyfriend.

Her therapist was interested in hearing what she meant by 'putting the past behind me', as this was a comment she had heard before from abuse survivors. Also, she hoped to learn more about her online life. Her goals were clear but needed to be SMART. So this is where they began, and agreed that Anita would think about how she would be different if these goals were achieved, so that they could talk about it next session.

Next time they met her therapist began by saying how great it was that Anita had been able to be so clear about the changes she wanted to make, and that she had decided to take time to talk about the impact her birthmark and the abuse were still having on her relationships. She noted that her goals identified changes she wanted to make in both these areas and wondered how or if these were connected. If the birthmark went away, would the relationship issues be improved or solved? After a moment Anita said not entirely, and they spent some time teasing apart the issues. Her cousin also had a visible difference and used a wheelchair, and she had wondered if that had something to do with why their uncle singled them out and thought he could silence them. She felt it would be hard to know whether or how her relationships would have been different, then added 'I guess if I felt better about myself and stronger it would have changed things'. Her therapist commented that her cosplay character was someone strong who could change things, and her blog gave her a space to say how she felt about abuse, so in this sense it was something she was already doing in these areas of her life. They talked about how she felt at those times, and the resources in these aspects of her self.

Considering this and looking at the notes Anita had made on her SMART goals it became clearer that both self-esteem and shame issues were influencing her current coping strategies. They talked again about the 'putting the past behind me' goal and her therapist felt it was helpful to work on the other issues first and see what impact that might have on how she thought and felt about this.

There are many ways this therapy episode could be approached. Anita has achieved a lot and has skills and resources to bring to the work, but any experienced therapist will see that there are some difficult issues to address, and realistic hopes to support so that she is not overwhelmed.

Anita has found CBT helpful in the past, and compassion focused work or ACT are also options. Her therapist also wonders about the times when she withdraws, crying alone, linking this with possible unresolved grief and trauma and shame. Again, the timeline 'maps' her journey so far, but can also be extended into the future, introducing the idea that the development of self is a process and she can return to some things later (for instance when she has a serious relationship).

A functional analysis helped them both to understand what was useful in her current coping pattern, and where there were opportunities for change. They discussed CBT and Compassion Focused approaches, and Anita chose to begin with developing a CBT for self-esteem formulation which she was familiar with.

While working on this her therapist also asked about her gaming 'avatar' and her cosplay identity, wondering what got in the way of connecting more with these aspects in other parts of her life. Anita thought that some people who knew her would be shocked to encounter this honest and assertive version. They also talked about who should 'own' any discriminatory behaviour which she did encounter, and how to take care of herself in those situations. Because of Anita's pattern of controlling situations (based on managing early life bullying) they also talked about negative assumptions she might be making and how to 'update' her coping in difficult encounters. This set the scene for planning some behavioural experiments, like mentioning her birthmark with good friends, not always wearing makeup (when away for a weekend, first thing in the morning), writing down her fears beforehand, and noting what really happened.

They referred back to the outline formulation they had started while planning these and talked about possible connections with her periods of crying.

Early experiences—impact of having a birthmark, and her uncle's abuse

Rules for Living—(identified through her current cognitive and behavioural coping strategies)—escape clauses, coping strategies, guidelines, policies, standards (Fig. 8.5).

Change methods—exposure for birthmark, schema work and role play. Giving herself permission to wear makeup, or not.

Relationships—allowing these to develop (criteria, standards), managing her anxiety (using situation analysis), ups and downs.

As part of their work on self-esteem Anita and her therapist discussed how her coping strategies limited her real intimacy in relationships (Erikson—intimacy vs. isolation) and the way in which managing this challenge was a normal developmental stage for young people. They

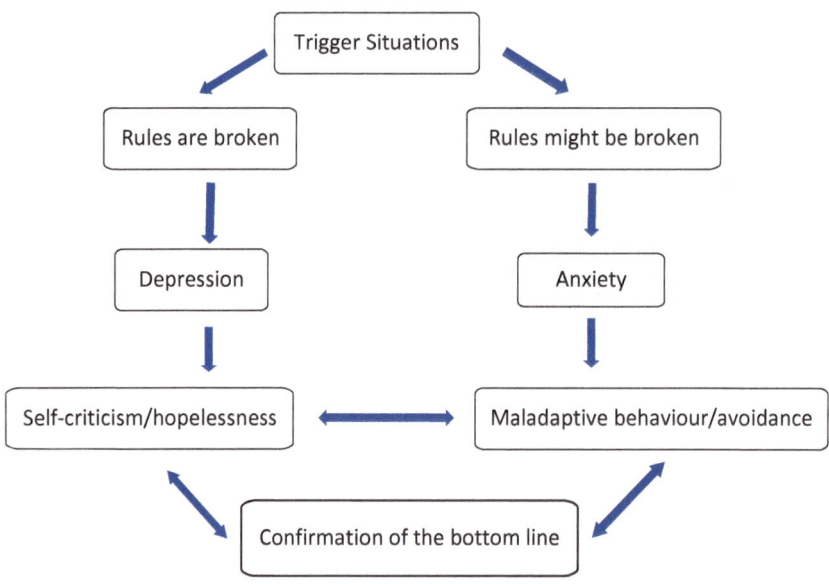

Fig. 8.5 Anita's 'Bottom Line' (schema, core belief) global negative self-judgement (or feared truth). Adapted from Lee (2009)

agreed that as Anita enjoyed writing a narrative task might be something that would be helpful, 'storying' herself to include all her selves and experience (privately), deciding what she wanted to share with her therapist and when. This proved to be a really important change method for her, especially when her therapist suggested that sharing the 'stuck' moments in the narrative would be useful. Anita did this, which is how her therapist first learned of the romantic bullying that had happened at university when a boyfriend used her anxieties to demean and control her. He was a 'catch' and Anita felt ashamed and paralysed, unable to deal with his temper and degrading comments. After escaping from this at the end of her course she vowed not to ever be in that situation again.

This disclosure was very helpful to the therapeutic conversation reflecting the level of trust that had developed. While talking this situation through they used the compassion-based formulation as a basis for thinking about her reactions, alternative ways of understanding her shame-based responses and supporting herself. This also led to revisions in her 'rules for living' and 'bottom line'.

Endnote—Anita is someone who found it very helpful to return to the same therapist when she began a more serious relationship, allowing her to work through real-time situations and behave differently, and draw on the work and materials created before.

References

Fennell MJV (1997) Low self esteem: A cognitive perspective. Behavioural and Cognitive Psychotherapy 25(1):1–25

Gilbert P (2010) The compassionate mind. Constable & Robinson, London

Lee D (2009) Compassion focused cognitive therapy for shame-based trauma memories and flashbacks in post-traumatic stress disorder. In: Grey N (ed) A casebook of cognitive therapy for traumatic stress reactions. Routledge, New York

Metcalf L (2004) The miracle question, answer it and change your life. Crown House Publishing

Sinclair M, Beadman M (2016) The little ACT workbook. Crimson Publishing Ltd, Bath

Some Final Thoughts

This book was begun in 2018 and completed in the summer of 2019/20. During that period there was a small trickle of online articles published on the experience of feeling different in a society increasingly entangled with social media, 'facetuning' apps and 'influencer' based marketing. This has been very useful for me as a writer. To balance this managed media output there is also more activity and connection via social media for people with visible difference and their families, potentially reducing their isolation (though this also attracts trolls at times). Still relatively few in number, these resources can easily be missed by those not affected or specifically interested, which is one reason why I have referred to some of them in this book. Disappointingly, though perhaps unsurprisingly, I also found a few examples of unfounded negative assumptions in both the media and research literature.

On the whole it is a hopeful time, and the possibility of a future in which we are all a bit more 'bionic' or genetically altered potentially changes the assumptions underlying social value. How you think this will turn out depends in part on whether you are fundamentally optimistic or pessimistic about the future. Are you able to share Stephen Pinker's view that we as a species are able to solve the significant challenges of climate

© The Author(s) 2020
V. Purcell, *Understanding Visible Differences*, Palgrave Texts in Counselling and Psychotherapy, https://doi.org/10.1007/978-3-030-51655-0

change and other things? Or that we are becoming more compassionate and less violent? (*Enlightenment Now* 2018).

The alternatives are not attractive. In the past, emerging from the Second World War, stigma and its medicalised reduction was a topic 'owned' by expert others, with limited input from those with lived experience. Goffman was writing about people who really needed to stay 'under the radar' to avoid abuse or worse. This is less true, though bullying and prejudice is still a problem. Organisations such as the NHS have a 'no decision about me, without me' rule and charities know that they need to include people 'living with' their issue. But even in this age of identity politics there is still a lingering sense of novelty in the idea that visibly different people might want loving relationships—hence the frisson behind 'The Undateables'.

Apart from these kinds of output there is an almost total absence of certain kinds of visible difference in mainstream media, reinforcing the implication that media careers are not suitable for certain types of people. If this seems extreme try to imagine a female newsreader with a facial difference (possibly one of the last taboos?). The absolute requirement that women on TV should be conventionally attractive to men at all times is (in my view) a measure of the distance that female emancipation still has to go. Keeping visibly different women in the backrooms is just a symptom of that. The unspoken message is—don't push it! In the UK Liz Cox is really an outlier in this respect, having established a career as an actor.

In 'Stigma' (1965) Goffman observed the 'rules of conduct' for those with differences, which included that they should always make the assumption that the other party 'meant well' even when they had (unintentionally?) caused offence. The responsibility for the safe management of interaction rested with the different other who must not confront or offend. Goffman's interest was in the people that society excluded, whether stigma was hidden, with sufferers attempting to 'pass', or obvious and inescapable.

The political and legal supports for diversity have altered the social climate somewhat (in some countries more than others). But progress is uneven and likely to remain so until we are truly freer and more equal. Things are better than ever, but there is much more to do! The importance of owning equal space and rights, despite persisting beauty preferences is the cutting edge of this effort. It is really extremely unlikely that people will stop preferring beauty, ableness and attractiveness over disfigurement and disability. But the unquestioned assumption that this preference automatically converts into favour, better jobs, more opportunities and so forth is one that could be challenged. The UK charity Changing Faces campaigns for facial equality. Face Equality Day was on 22 May 2019 and promotes the idea that everyone should be treated fairly and equally, whatever the appearance of their face and body. My guess is that it went largely un-noticed by the majority of the country.

For clinicians, a target audience for this book, I have wanted to emphasise the importance of seeing the social/cultural and religious context of their clients' lives when attempting to understand their experience. It is not enough to tick the 'social anxiety' box and run the protocol. Your client's mental health and wellbeing outcomes depend crucially on not internalizing social prejudice. A tough job on a bad day, they need to be connected with supportive others. Among your clients there may also be those who have been too skilful in constructing lives which avoid social harms, limiting their choices un-necessarily in the process. You could help them see this and build more challenging and rewarding lives. This is the way that things will change. In this respect some aspects of identity politics are very helpful and a lot of intellectual heavy lifting has been done in the 'struggle'. I personally would not wish people with visible differences to be seen as 'yet another victim group'. Remaining in separate 'silos' of difference (even if they are comfortable ones) can only go so far.

I have deliberately made the category of visible difference wide to include people who are able-bodied but look different as well as those disabled. Because of the unique psychological aspects of 'passing' and feeling that you don't I have specifically not included: hidden differences and body dysmorphia. These are very important topics which require more space to do them justice.

I hope you as a reader find something here which helps your practice and your experience.

Reference

Pinker S (2018) *Enlightenment Now.* Penguin Books Ltd/Viking

Appendix: Brief Summary of Types of Visible Difference

Two Main Categories

Differences at Birth (Congenital)

A congenital condition is defined as one which existed pre-memory (Harris 1997), meaning that the individual has no experience of what life might be like without their condition. They may in some cases be linked with cognitive impairments and other medical problems which influence the degree of impact.

Some conditions are present at birth but become less visible over time following treatment, for instance haemangiomas (non-cancerous growths of the blood vessels). Others such as neurofibromatosis, which is a genetic condition causing tumours to form on nerve tissue, and characterized by brown spots on the skin, have the opposite pattern. Kleinfelter's syndrome, in which male children have an extra x chromosome is another.

Harris (1997) classifies congenital conditions according to the type or affected body type, and the following listings are not comprehensive. When working with a client who has a visible difference the therapist is advised to do their own research to ensure their understanding of the condition is sufficient, as well as enquiring about the patient's own

© The Author(s) 2020
V. Purcell, *Understanding Visible Differences*, Palgrave Texts in Counselling and Psychotherapy, https://doi.org/10.1007/978-3-030-51655-0

experience. This will avoid tedious questioning of the patient. It may also be that there are aspects of their treatment they do not fully recall, but which might be relevant, and others they regard as unique to them, but which are common experiences for others with the same condition. This is more likely to be true of an older person who has had little peer support.

It is also worth noting that the World Health Organisation (2015) estimates that globally 303,000 newborns die within four weeks due to congenital abnormalities. Ninety-four per cent of congenital abnormalities occur in low- and middle-income countries, with socio-economics, infection and environment all cited as factors. Consanguinity (where parents are blood relatives) increases the prevalence of rare congenital abnormalities, and smaller populations such as Ashkenazi Jews have a comparatively higher proportion of genetic mutations such as haemophilia and cystic fibrosis.

Craniofacial Conditions

These involve the head and neck and can be numerous and varied. They are classified as either anomalous, a malformation or a sequence (Billaud Feragen 2012). An anomalous defect is a structural or functional deficit present at birth. A malformation is the result of incorrect morphogenesis, and a sequence is a series of defects which occur in a nonrandom way. Examples of sequences are Pierre Robin Sequence where the child has a small lower jaw and tongue that falls back into the throat, along with breathing difficulties. Also, DiGeorge Sequence which is caused by the deletion of a small sequence of chromosome 22. Symptoms can be variable and involve many organs as well as facial defects. Goldenhar Syndrome is a rare example of a sequence, which causes incomplete development of the ear, nose, soft palate, lip and mandible.

The most common anomalous craniofacial condition is a cleft of lip/ and/or palate, found in approximately 1–2 per 1000 newborns (Silvertsen et al. 2008). It is caused by a disruption of the process of cell fusion during facial development in the 5th–11th weeks of gestation. Timing of the disturbance affects laterality and degree of severity. The causes are still not fully understood but involve interactions of genetic and environmental factors, and may sometimes be associated with other anomalies (Jugessur and Murray 2005).

There are a wide range of other conditions involving the head and neck, all comparatively rare. For instance, hemifacial microsomias are failures of part of the head and neck to develop. Treacher Collins syndrome causes the underdevelopment of the cheek and jawbones, or there may be complex facial clefts with missing features which will require surgical reconstruction.

Congenital Conditions Involving the Nervous System

These are birth defects which occur during foetal intrauterine growth and affect the physical structure of the brain or spinal cord. This broad term covers a wide range of disorders and medical conditions from minor to severe, including spina bifida (in which the spinal cord does not form properly), or microcephaly in which brain growth is inhibited. Some of these abnormalities are caused by genetic factors. In other cases, exposure to one or more multifactorial influences is the cause for instance—alcohol, smoking, drugs, vitamins, medications, environmental toxins, virus or other toxic substances which can affect the baby in the womb and contribute to the development of an abnormality in the central nervous system. In many infants no identifiable cause is found however.

Congenital Conditions Involving Vascular Development

This category can be divided into vascular tumours or haemangiomas, and vascular malformations. Haemangiomas mainly occur in a visible location on the head and neck, proliferating between the ages of 6 and 10 months, and disappear completely before the child is 10 years old. Vascular malformations such as port wine stains are less common, are present at birth and do not fade or disappear.

Congenital Conditions Involving Other Body Parts

The prevalence of these conditions is the same as those involving the head and neck. This category includes the failure of part of a limb to develop, and shape anomalies, like syndactyly which is the failure of fingers and toes to separate, polydactyly which causes the growth of extra digits, and clubfoot.

Dwarfism is a term applied to conditions resulting in unusually short stature which can have complex causes. Signs and symptoms are often present at birth or in early infancy. The most common types are skeletal dysplasias which are genetic, but many people of restricted height have two parents in the normal height range. Dwarfism may also become visible later during the course of a child's development. It can be caused by bone growth disorders, or hormone disorders, and as such it may sometimes belong in the following category of acquired difference.

Acquired Physical Differences

Accidents and Burns

While it is hoped that advances in our understanding of genetics and increased prosperity may eventually prevent some congenital disorders, acquired differences are likely to remain part of human experience. They occur in two main categories: either as the result of injury, trauma and disease, or caused by medical interventions which are appearance altering. Traumas causing injury could include road traffic accidents, violent attacks, industrial accidents and burns caused by fire or chemicals. These, plus surgery and other invasive treatment regimes may mean that the person's sense of who they are in the world is suddenly and dramatically altered in a way they experience as entirely negative.

Improvements in the treatment of burns and other traumatic injuries mean that people are able to survive more extensive injuries across all age groups. Wisley and Gaskell (2012) report that burn injuries are experienced by 250,000 people in the UK each year, the majority being the result of scalds or flames. Most cover less than 10% of the body. There is a gender imbalance in this form of trauma, with males outnumbering females, and they occur more frequently among those who are psychologically vulnerable (Klinge et al. 2009). Researchers report more risk-taking behaviours in this group, and among children a higher prevalence of ADHD and ADD. The most challenging group to support psychologically are those who have self-immolated.

The extensive treatment now offered often means a lengthy and painful road to recovery, at the end of which they are likely to have challenges in adjustment. Research again shows that the severity of the injury does not predict difficulty, and other personality and social support factors are important. James Partridge, one of the founders of the charity Changing Faces and himself the survivor of severe facial burns, has suggested that recovery from burns involves moving through several stages (Partridge 2005). The focus in the first stage is on survival and the physical aspects of recovery and rehabilitation. Post discharge, the transition from a pre-burn identity to a self that has a permanent disfigurement must be achieved, and he identifies a third stage as 'advocacy' in which a sense of self not organized around a social ideal of attractiveness is formed, rebuilding self-esteem on different foundations. It hardly needs to be said that this is a difficult and significant achievement in a society focused on physical appearance. This psychological journey will be explored further in the chapters on treatment.

Differences Associated with Disease and Illness

Other acquired visible differences associated with disease and illness occur at different stages of life, each presenting challenge for the family, partners and individual depending on the circumstances. For example, acne which can affect any age group but is much more common in adolescence. It is thought to be stimulated by increases in testosterone and other sex hormones and affects twice as many males as females. While acne can occur in up to 85% of young people in adolescence (Balkrishnan et al. 2006) it usually disappears in young adulthood. Rarer and more severe forms include the formation of cysts which can result in permanent scarring. Purvis et al. (2006) in a large study of young people in New Zealand found that psychological distress increased in relation to severity, with a higher incidence of suicidal thoughts and attempts.

Eczema usually first appears in childhood, with most present before the age of 5. Pressures on the family caused by stress, sleep deprivation and interruption to employment can be serious, and children are more likely to be teased and bullied at school. Family based interventions can help them cope, but these are currently very limited. Eczema usually clears by the age of 16, but in cases where it persists through adolescence there may be an equal pattern of distress to acne at a stage of life when appearance becomes more important. Stress has a role in the inflammatory process, but few evidence-based treatment programmes are available at any stage as the research is yet to be conducted (Bundy 2012).

Vitiligo is characterised by a progressive development of scattered white patches of skin due to loss of pigment cells, and it occurs in approximately 1% of the population. Multiple causative factors are involved, though approximately one-fifth of sufferers have a relative with the condition. It occurs with similar frequency in all ethnic groups though it is more visible with dark skin, and it is generally considered to be an autoimmune disease.

Psoriasis is a heritable chronic inflammatory condition mediated by immune system function, and it is characterised by excessive growth and shedding of the upper layers of the skin. It usually emerges in adulthood. When active it is visible and distressing but has a pattern of flare-ups and periods of remission. It is complex to manage, often occurring alongside other conditions like arthritis and Crohn's disease. It is well recognised as a disfiguring and stigmatizing skin disease, and sufferers report distress, shame, embarrassment and psychological burden (Kimball et al. 2010) particularly if it is visible on the face.

Though this is not intended to be a comprehensive list it is worth mentioning stroke, which although uncommon in young adults can be a traumatic and isolating illness. They comprise 10–15% of all stroke patients, and there are over 1.2 million stroke survivors in the UK. The physical challenges that occur post-stroke if it is not treated quickly can include paralysis of parts of the body, facial and movement problems, and visual and speech problems. Some of the psychological difficulties mentioned so far also apply to this group though little specialist help is available post discharge.

Differences Following Surgical and Medical Treatments

These interventions can result in scarring or disfigurement to different degrees where the focus is on saving maximum function or life. The psychological impact of these changes can be difficult to predict, as it depends on the adjustment of the individual and may not be related to severity. However surgical amputation, head and neck surgery, breast cancer surgery and stoma formation are recognised as four specialist fields that can dramatically alter body image (Williamson et al. 2010).

Horgan and MachLachlan (2004) offer considerable evidence of social stigma and interpersonal difficulties after lower limb amputation, some of which are caused by the embarrassment or patronising behaviour of others. Positive adjustment to amputation is more likely for those with a pre-existing optimistic disposition and active coping skills. For those who do not have these advantages, therapy and social skills training to manage the reactions of others can be helpful.

Surgery for head and neck cancer can result in scarring, changes in facial shape, drooling, paralysis and difficulty with eating and speaking. All patients will experience some permanent appearance change and Semple et al. (2004) report that anxiety and depression are experienced by 30–40% (which seems low) and can continue to escalate post treatment.

The outcome of different surgical and reconstruction options for breast cancer has been the subject of considerable research (for instance Nano et al. 2005), which informs us that women who survive and undergo breast conserving surgery or immediate reconstructive surgery are likely to retain a more positive body image and report fewer appearance concerns. Satisfaction with the cosmetic result is more important than the type of surgery. The degree of investment in physical appearance and the value placed on specific body parts predict success in adaptation post surgery.

An abdominal stoma is a permanent or temporary opening in the abdomen which is connected to a bag (usually) designed to collect faecal or urinary waste. Appliances can normally be hidden under clothes, but even one that is functioning well requires closer contact with waste and smells, which are tolerated less well by some patients. They report distressing changes in body image and a reluctance towards physical closeness with others. This alteration in the experience of self, allied with fears of disgusting others, is more likely to be felt by women than men.

In addition to these, the physical changes wrought by medical treatments like chemotherapy and anti-retroviral therapy are recognized as being likely to cause negative changes to appearance. It hardly needs to be said that the individual patient is undergoing these at a time when they have few resources not already fully challenged by the treatment. In rare cases the prospect of hair loss and weight gain can lead patients to refuse treatment and hide their illness until it is too late (Williamson et al. 2010).

References

Balkrishnan R, Kulkarni AS, Cayce K, Feldman SR (2006) Predictors of health-care outcomes and costs related to medication use in patients with acne in the United States. Cutis 77(4):251–255

Billaud Feragen K (2012) Congenital conditions. In: Rumsey N, Harcourt D (eds) Oxford handbook of the psychology of appearance. Oxford University Press

Bundy C (2012) Visible difference associated with disease: skin conditions. In: Rumsey N, Harcourt D (eds) Oxford handbook of the psychology of appearance. Oxford University Press

Harris D (1997) Types, causes, and physical treatment of visible differences. In: Lansdown R, Rumsey N, Bradbury E, Carr A, Partridge J (eds) Visibly different: coping with disfigurement. Butterworth-Heinemann, Oxford, pp 79–90

Horgan O, MachLachlan M (2004) Psychosocial adjustment to lower limb amputation: a review. Disabil Rehabil 26(14/15):837–850

Jugessur A, Murray JC (2005) Orofacial clefting: recent insights into a complex trait. Curr Opin Genet Dev 15:270–278

Kimball AB, Gieler U, Linder D, Sampogna F, Warren RB, Augustin M (2010) Psoriasis: is the impairment to a patient's life cumulative? J Acad Dermatol Venereol 24:987–1004

Klinge K, Chamberlain DJ, Redden M, King L (2009) Psychological adjustments made by post-burn injury patients: an integrative literature review. J Adv Nurs 65:2274–2292

Nano MT, Gill PG, Kollias J, Bochner M A, Malycha P, Winefeld HR (2005) Psychological impact and cosmetic outcome of surgical breast cancer strategies. ANZ J Sur 75(11):940–947

Partridge J (2005) Changing faces: the challenge of facial disfigurement. Penguin, London

Purvis D, Robinson E, Merry S, Watson P (2006) Acne, anxiety, depression and suicide in teenagers: a cross-sectional survey of New Zealand secondary school sudents. J Paediatr Child Health 42(12):793–796

Semple CJ, Sullivan K, Dunwoody L, Kernohan G (2004) Psychosocial interventions for patients with head and neck cancer. Cancer Nurs 27(6):434–444

Silvertsen A, Wilcox A, Johnson GE, Abyholm F, Vindenes HA, Lie RT (2008) Prevalence of major anatomical variations in oral clefts. Plast Reconstr Surg 121:587–595

Williamson H, Harcourt D, Halliwell E, Frith H, Wallace M (2010) Adolescents and parents experiences of managing the psychosocial consequences of an altered appearance during treatment for cancer. J Pediatr Oncol Nurs 27(3):168–175

Wisley J, Gaskell S (2012) The Oxford handbook of the psychology of appearance 372–398. Oxford University Press

Resources Support and Information

Achondroplasia.co.uk
Support and information for those with short limb dwarfism, their families and carers.
Tel 01761 471 257
Website: www.achondroplasia.co.uk
Alopecia Patient's Society—Hairline International
Help and support for people with alopecia and all hair loss conditions.
Website: www.hairlineinternational.com
Arthritis Care
Support and information for people with any form of arthritis.
Tel Helpline 0808 800 4050
Website: www.arthritiscare.org.uk
The Arthrogryposis Group (TAG)
Support and advice for those with this condition.
Tel 01299 825 781
Website: www.tagonline.org.uk
The Birthmark Support Group
A support group for people with birthmarks.
Tel 0845 045 4700

© The Author(s) 2020
V. Purcell, *Understanding Visible Differences*, Palgrave Texts in Counselling and
Psychotherapy, https://doi.org/10.1007/978-3-030-51655-0

Website: www.birthmarksupportgroup.org.uk
Breast Cancer Care
Support, information and advice to those diagnosed with or recovering from breast cancer.
Tel 0808 800 6000
Website: www.breastcancercare.org.uk
British Allergy Foundation
Information service for people with all types of allergies, including skin allergies.
Tel 0208 303 8583
Website: www.allergyuk.org
British Association of Dermatologists
Information on dermatological conditions.
Tel 0207 383 0266
Website: www.bad.org.uk
British Association of Skin Camouflage
Training, advice and assistance.
Tel 01226 790744
Website:skin-camouflage.net
British Red Cross Skin Camouflage Service
Helpline 0300 012 0276
Website: http://redcross.org.uk/what-we-do/Health-and-social-care/skin-camouflage
Burns Centre Care Katie Piper Foundation : https://katiepiperfoundation.org.uk/
Website: http://www.burncentrecare.co.uk/support.html
Children's Burns Trust (CBT)
Offers information and advice to burn and scald injured children and their families.
Website: www.cbtrust.org.uk
Changing Faces—Based in London, a UK charity offering resources and support for people with disfigurements of the face and body. Campaigns. Schools training support.
Tel 0845 4500 275
Website: http//www.changingfaces.org.uk

Cleft Lip and Palate Association (CLAPA)
Website: www.clapa.com
DebRa
Helpline—01344 771961
Website: www.debra.org.uk
Travelling specialist nurses, financial help and respite for people with epidermolysis bullosa (EB). Also funds research into EB.
Different Strokes
Local peer support groups for younger stroke survivors and their carers.
Tel 0345 130 7172 or 01908 317 618
Website: www.differentstrokes.co.uk
Ehlers-Danlos Support Group
Website: www.ehlers-danlos.org
Information, support and advice.
Facial Palsy UK
Support groups, campaigns and information for those with this and related conditions, families and friends.
Tel 0300 030 9333
Website: www.facialpalsy.org.uk
Ichthyosis Support Group
Website: http://www.ichthyosis.org.uk.
Information network and support system for affected children and adults.
Let's Face It
Tel—01843 833724
Website: www.lets-face-it.org.uk.
Information and support for people with facial differences and their families.
Limbless Association
Helpline—01277725182
Website: www.limbless-association.org
Offers information, advice and support to the limbless community.
Lymphoedema Support Network
Website: www.lymphodema.org/Index.asp
Information and support to patients with lymphedema.
National Ankylosing Spondylitis Society

Tel 01435 873527

Website: www.nass.co.uk

A forum for patients, as well as information and advice for those with AS.

National Eczema Society

Helpline 0870 271 3604

Website: www.eczema.org

Support and advice for people with eczema.

National Lichen Sclerosus Support Group (UK)

Website: www.lichensclerosus.org

Information and support for lichen sclerosus.

Neurofibromatosis Association

Helpline 0208 439 1234

Website: www.nfauk.org

Support, advice and help for people with neurofibromatosis.

Nevus Outreach

Website: www.nevus.org

Psoriasis and Psoriatic Arthritis Alliance (PAPAA)

Website: www.papaa.org

UK registered charity for people affected by psoriasis and psoriatic arthritis.

Psoriasis Forum

Website: www.psoriasis-help.org.uk

Interactive forum offering support groups for sufferers.

Psoriasis Association

Helpline 01604 711129

Website: timewarp.demon.co.uk/psoriasis.html

Advice, help and support.

Raynaud's Scleroderma Association

Tel 01270 872766

Website: www.raynauds.org.uk

Information and support for people affected by Raynaud's and scleroderma.

Stroke Association

Website: www.stroke.org.uk

National organisation with local branches. Fundraising, volunteering, research, local support groups and supporter care.

The Thyroid Eye Disease Charitable Trust
Tel 0844 800 8133
Website: www.stuartchadwick.me.uk/TED/index.html,
Information and support. Also offers a network of support groups.

UK Craniofacial Support Group
Tel 01454 850557
Website: www.headlines.org.uk
Support and advice for people with any form of craniofacial condition or syndrome.

Vitiligo Society
Helpline 0207 840 0855. Website: www.vitigliosociety.org.uk
Information and support for people with vitiligo.

Xeroderma Pigmentosum (XP) Support Group
Helpline 01494 890981
Website: www.xpsupportgroup.org.uk
Support, help and information for this and other photosensitive conditions.

Index

A

Aaron Beck 1979, 109
Abuse, 99
Acquired Difference, 44
ACT formulation, 137
Act of 'Passing', 12
Adam Pearson, 24
Adolescence & social media, 87
Adolescent transition, 49
African Child Policy Forum, x
Akhenaten, 11
Alita battleangel, 149
Altabe and Thompson 1996, 28
Anita (case study), 148–153
Antenatal diagnosis & support, 34
Appearance anxiety and shame, 101
'Appearance related' conversation–
    Jones 2018, 67
'Appearance related' distress, 20
Arteriovenous malformation, 25
Assessment tools, 100

Attachment, facially different
    babies, 36
Attractiveness bias, 36
Augustus-Horvath and Tylka
    2009, 99
Avoidance, 121

B

Barlow & Ellard 2006, 62
Bateson 2002, 13
Baumrind (1991–attachment &
    parenting, 40
Bearman 2006, 39
Beavers and Hampson (2003), 65
Bellew (2012), 60
Berry 2000, ix
'Beauty is good' stereotype, 37
Bes, 11
Bigorexia, 101
Black et al 2013, 123

© The Author(s) 2020
V. Purcell, *Understanding Visible Differences*, Palgrave Texts in Counselling and
Psychotherapy, https://doi.org/10.1007/978-3-030-51655-0

Body Dysmorphia, 9
Body Esteem-Harter 2003, Stice and
    Bearman 2001, 66
Bordin 1979, 105
Boudicca Fox-Leonard 2018, 91–92
Bourdieu's (1986)-body as social
    capital, 48
Brown 2012, 34
Brune & Wilson 2013, 12
Building resilience, 71–73
Bullying, 63–65
Bullying at school-Vannatta 2009,
    Bradbury 1997, 79–80
Burn Camps, 47
Butler 2015, 43

C
Cadogan 2010, 48
Camp 2002, 103
Carter and McGoldrick 1988, 72
CBT Formulation, 135
Changing Faces Survey, 91
Charles VI, 11
Children's story books, 78
Clarke 2009, 102
Clarke 2014, 122
Cognitive processing models, 28
Compassion focus–Gilbert 2009, 109
Compassion focussed
    formulation, 136
Congenital defect, 8
Coping skills, 39, 40
Cyberbullying, 90

D
Dealing with intrusive comments, 82
Development of Self, 43

Differences–Congenital &
    Acquired, 71
Disability Discrimination Act
    1995, 22
Dittmar and Halliwell 2008, 28
Diversity training, 78
Doorknob moments, 115
Dwarfism, 11, 25

E
Ecological systems
    theory–Bronfenbrenner
    1992, 106
Egan 2011, 53
Elizabeth Day 2014, 24
Erikson, 44, 49, 50
Erving Goffman 1963, 8
Eugene Grant–Street abuse, 38
Evolutionary psychology, 13
External Shame, 102

F
Facial burns & adjustment–Blakeney
    1988, 67
Facial port wine stain, 148
Faith & spirituality, 61
Falvey 2012, 12
F D Roosevelt, 12
Festinger's Social Comparison
    Theory (1954), 27
Formulation, 133
Frederickson 1997, 9
Frisen and Holmqvist 2010, 39
Functional analysis, 99
Functional contextualism-Vilardaga
    and Hayes 2009, 107
Functional Impairment, 16

G

Gergen 1985, 13
Gilbert & Andrews 1998, 102
Gilbert and Miles 2002,
    102–103

H

Harvard's Pluralism project, 59
Healthy family systems, 63
Honour based cultures, ix
Hopkins 2011, 27
Hoss and Langlois
    (2003)–Averaging
    hypothesis, 36

I

Internalised fear of difference, 8
Internet resources, 64
Intersectionality–Crenshaw
    1991, 43
Irving 1990, 28
Irwin et al 2016, 101

J

James Partridge 1990, 46
J James (case study), 143–148
Johanssen and Ringsberg
    (2004), 35
Johnson 2012, x

K

Katie Piper, 48
Katy's Story, 28
Kent & Thompson 2002, 8
Kish and Lansdown 2000, 83

L

Lansdown 1997, 41
Levinson 1986, 72
Lewis 2003, 99
Liz Carr 2006, 89
Lowes and Tiggemann
    (2003)-Observer
    perspective, 45
Loss of privacy, x

M

Mary Douglas 1966, ix
Men & Chicken 2015, 20
Mentalisation-based approach, 86
'Miracle question,' 137, 145
Multicultural, ix

N

Narrative work for multiple
    trauma-Schauer 2011, 125
Nelson 1994, 19
NHS outpatient therapy, 84
Nikki Lilly, 25
Non-stigmatising explanations, 61

O

Objectification Theory-Frederickson
    and Roberts 1997, 8, 98
O'Connor 2018, 79
O'Dell and Prior 2004, 86
Older Adults & romantic
    relationships, 54
Older Women study–Piran
    2017, 52
Ong 2007, 53
Orbach S 2009, 13

P

Paralympics, 22
Parental rejection-Rohner
    2008, 68
Pat Barker (2012), 18
Paul Longmore (2003), 19
Peer relationships, 66
Personhood, 33
Perspective, 13
Peter Dinklage, 25
Piran's Developmental Theory of
    Embodiment (2017), 50
PLISSIT model-Clarke 2014, 96
Post-traumatic growth–Calhoun
    2010, 126
Protecting the professional self–
    Harte Bratt 2019, 124–125
Psychological trauma, 47, 99
PTSD–Corry 2010, 47

R

Ramsay and Langlois (2002), 37
Readiness for change–Prochaska
    1992, 110–111
Ready Player One–Spielberg–Ernest
    Cline, 26
Reciprocal resonance, 124
Relatives' shameful feelings-Rossi
    2005, Kornhaber 2018,
    71–72
Resilience-Lia and Abela 2016, 71
Resources for schools, 83
Restricted Growth Association, 39
Robinson 1997, 66
Rolland 2018, 103
Romance, 90
Rumsey and Harcourt 2017, 66

S

Sarah (case study), 139–143
Scaffolding, 49
Self-esteem–Argyle (2008), 41
Self objectification theory-
    Frederickson and Roberts
    (1997), 46
Severe disfigurements, 22
Sexual abuse, 24
Shaffer 2000, 13
Shame, 99–103
Shaw Trust, 22
Sibling issues, 61–62
Smith 2012, 87
Smolak (2010, 2012), 37
Social Constructionist, 13
Social skills training, 30
Soft Prejudice, 79
'Spoiled Identity', 8
Social graces (John Burnham
    2012), 44
Social Media Victimisation, 14
Social 'norming,' 27
Social stigma & disability-Rolland
    2018, 69
Specialist support groups, 85
Stanley 1963, 26
Starting school, 77
Stereotypes of 'Difference', 14
Stigma, 17
Stigma consciousness, 103
'Struggle for rights', 21
Supervision relationship–Jones
    2003, 124
Support groups, 81
Supportive reciprocal resonance
    Dallos and Vetere 2009, 126
Surgical interventions (impact of), 83

Systemic Formulation-Dallos and
    Draper 2015, 107
Systemic stance, 132
Systemic stance-Fonagy and Bateman
    2006, 107

Termination, severe foetal
    handicap, 34
Terminations and disability, x
Therapeutic alliance-Horvath and
    Bedi 2002, Baldwin 2007, 105
Therapeutic colonisation-Per Jensen
    2016, 120
Therapeutic letters-Kindsvatter
    2013, 69
Therapeutic relationship-Kazantzis
    2017, Lavender 2019, 109
Thompson and Kent Objectification
    Theory, 98
Time line, 99
Tonks, Henry, 18
Toxic shame–Tomkins 1963, 100
Tuchman 1971, 18
Tulsi Vajani 2020, 15
Tutankhamun, 11
Typological Approach, 7
Tyrion, Game of Thrones, 97

The Undateables, 24
University Counselling, 74
Use of Time & Timelines,
    115–116

Vermaes 2012, 62
Vilardaga 2007, 108
Visibly different (meaning of), 1–9

Walsh 2012, 60–61
Walsh 2016, 65
Weilage and Hope (1999), 46
Wheeler and Miyake 1992, 28
Widdows 2018, 13
Withdrawal & avoidance, 86
Womens' Activism, 18
Womens' Suffrage, 14
Wonder 2017, 62
Wood 1994, 18

Young adulthood–moving
    away, 89